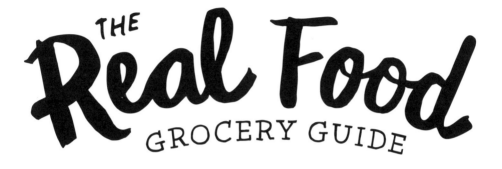

THE Real Food
GROCERY GUIDE

Navigate the Grocery Store • Ditch Artificial and

Unsafe Ingredients • Bust Nutritional Myths

• Select the Healthiest Foods Possible

MARIA MARLOWE, C.H.C.

FAIR WINDS

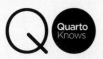

Quarto is the authority on a wide range of topics.

Quarto educates, entertains and enriches the lives of our readers—enthusiasts and lovers of hands-on living.

www.QuartoKnows.com

First published in the United States of America in 2017 by Fair Winds Press, an imprint of Quarto Publishing Group USA Inc.
100 Cummings Center
Suite 265-D
Beverly, Massachusetts 01915-6101
Telephone: (978) 282-9590
Fax: (978) 283-2742
QuartoKnows.com
Visit our blogs at QuartoKnows.com

21 20 19 18 17   1 2 3 4 5

ISBN: 978-1-59233-755-2

Digital edition published in 2017.

Names: Marlowe, Maria, author.
Title: The real food grocery guide : navigate the grocery store, ditch
   artificial & unsafe ingredients, bust nutritional myths & select the
   healthiest foods possible / Maria Marlowe, C.H.C.
Description: Beverly, Massachusetts : Quarto Publishing Group USA, Inc.,
   [2017] | Includes bibliographical references and index.
Identifiers: LCCN 2016046012 | ISBN 9781592337552 (trade pbk.)
Subjects: LCSH: Grocery shopping. | Natural foods.
Classification: LCC TX356 .M385 2017 | DDC 641.3/02--dc23
LC record available at https://lccn.loc.gov/2016046012

Design and Page Layout: Debbie Berne
Cover Image: Glenn Scott Photography
Photography: Glenn Scott Photography and Shutterstock

Printed in China

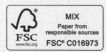

MIX
Paper from responsible sources
FSC® C016973
www.fsc.org

The information in this book is for educational purposes only. It is not intended to replace the advice of a physician or medical practitioner. Please see your health care provider before beginning any new health program.

To anyone who has ever been confused about what to eat.

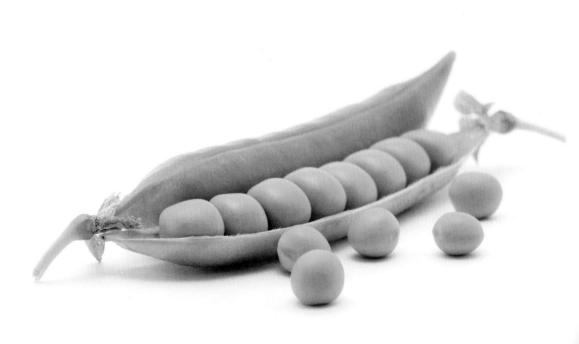

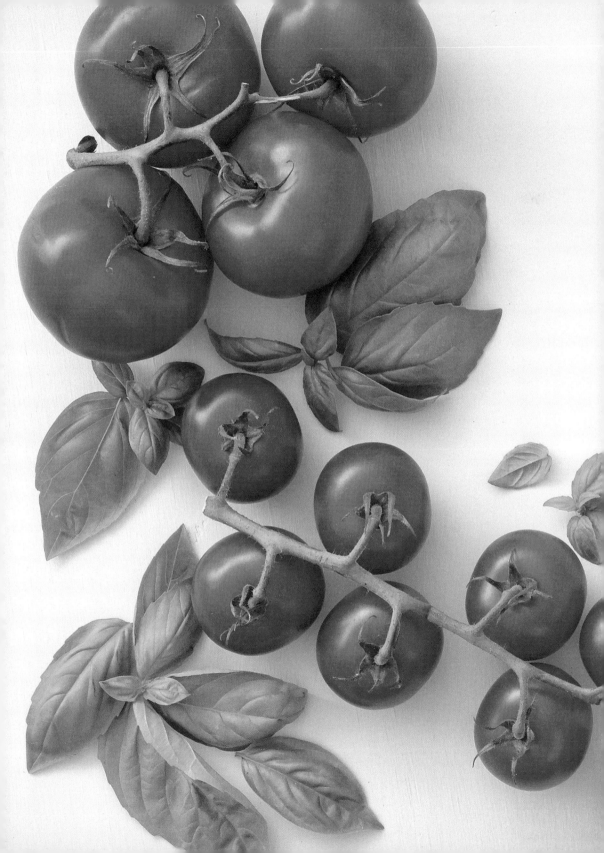

CONTENTS

FOREWORD

Many people are interested in eating healthier, but making such a big change can sometimes feel overwhelming.

Wouldn't it be great if you had a trusted field guide who could take you by the hand and walk you through every aisle of the grocery store, explain the health benefits and concerns of each food group, and then offer tips for selecting the best, most nutritious variety of each?

Well, now you do. It's in your hands—literally and figuratively.

The Real Food Grocery Guide is one of the most practical and user-friendly books I've ever seen about navigating your way through a new way of eating and living. Maria Marlowe shows you how and why a whole foods, plant-based diet is the healthiest way to eat.

For almost four decades, my colleagues and I at the nonprofit Preventive Medicine Research Institute and the University of California, San Francisco, have conducted clinical research proving the **many benefits of comprehensive lifestyle changes**. These include the following:

- A whole foods, plant-based diet

- Stress management techniques, including yoga and meditation

- Moderate exercise, such as walking

- Social support and community (love and intimacy)

In short—eat well, move more, stress less, and love more.

Many people tend to think of advances in medicine as high-tech and expensive, such as a new drug, laser, or surgical procedure. We often have a hard time believing that something as simple as comprehensive lifestyle changes can make such a powerful difference in our lives—but they often do.

In our research, we've used high-tech, expensive, state-of-the-art scientific measures to prove the power of these simple, low-tech, low-cost interventions. These randomized controlled trials and other studies have been published in the leading peer-reviewed medical and scientific journals.

In addition to *preventing* many chronic diseases, these lifestyle changes can often *reverse* the progression of these illnesses. In all our studies, we found that the more people changed their diet and lifestyle, the more their conditions improved and the better they felt—at any age. It's not all or nothing: If you indulge yourself one day, just eat healthier the next.

In our research, we showed for the first time that lifestyle changes alone can reverse the progression of even severe coronary heart disease. There was even more reversal after five years than after one year and two and a half times fewer cardiac events. We also found that these lifestyle changes can reverse type 2 diabetes and may slow, stop, or even reverse the progression of early stage prostate cancer.

What's more, changing your lifestyle actually changes your genes, turning on genes that keep you healthy and turning off genes that promote heart disease, prostate cancer, breast cancer, and diabetes—more than five hundred genes in only three months. Our latest research found that these diet and lifestyle changes may even lengthen telomeres, the ends of your chromosomes that control aging: As your telomeres get longer, your life gets longer.

And what's good for you is good for our planet, too. Transitioning toward a whole foods plant-based diet not only makes a difference in our own lives, it also makes a difference in the lives of many others across the globe.

Here's why: Many people are surprised to learn that animal agribusiness generates more greenhouse gases than all forms of transportation combined. More than half of the grain produced in the United States and nearly 40 percent of the world's grain is fed to livestock rather than consumed directly by humans. In the United States, more than eight billion livestock are maintained, which eat about seven times the amount of grain consumed by the entire population.

It takes about ten times as much energy to eat a meat-based diet versus a plant-based diet. Producing 2.2 pounds (1 kg) of fresh beef requires about 29 pounds (13 kg) of grain and 66 pounds (30 kg) of forage. This much grain and forage requires a total of 11,350 gallons (43,000 L) of water.

So, when we choose to eat a plant-based diet, we free up tremendous amounts of resources that can benefit many others as well as ourselves. We do have enough food in the world to feed everyone—if only enough people were to eat lower on the food chain. I find this very meaningful. And when we can act more compassionately, it helps our hearts as well.

—Dean Ornish, M.D.

Founder and president, Preventive Medicine Research Institute, clinical professor of medicine, University of California, San Francisco, and author, *The Spectrum* and *Dr. Dean Ornish's Program for Reversing Heart Disease*

www.ornish.com

LETTER FROM THE AUTHOR

What are you eating?

Most of the time, we only ask this question when we spot a loved one eating something that looks delicious, in hopes that our feigned curiosity will result in being offered a bite.

But I implore you to ask yourself—and your family—the same question from a more serious perspective. It's a question I wish someone had asked me back in 2002. It would have saved me five years of self-imposed food-induced misery.

Here's how it started. Right after my sixteenth birthday—the day after my Sweet Sixteen to be exact—I woke up with a red bump the size of a small mountain on my chin. The next day, a second one appeared—then another and another. So I grabbed some acne cream and started to play a game of whack-a-mole on my face. Just as I'd get one zit to shrink, another one (or three) would pop up.

Before long, my face was covered in acne and started to resemble the pizza I so loved to eat. The adults told me it was my age—a teenage rite of passage. But that justification didn't sit well with me, especially as my older brother and younger sister—only a couple years apart from me—were largely unscathed by this so-called "teenage" dilemma.

I tried every lotion under the sun. I saw multiple dermatologists and was even prescribed Accutane. It came with a laundry list of side effects—including severe depression, which could lead to suicide—so I decided not to try it and resigned myself to the fact that I was simply cursed. Clearly, I thought, my affliction must have been caused by bad genes, bad luck, or bad karma.

But if my acne hadn't become so severe that I eventually refused to leave the house, this book may have never come to fruition. Even though it tormented me through high school and parts of college, my acne turned out to be a blessing in disguise because it sparked my journey into the world of food and nutrition.

Along the way, I realized that our bodies do a good job of telling us what they need—if we're only willing to listen. It turned out that my acne wasn't the result of bad genes, bad luck, or bad karma—it was simply the result of a bad diet. Until that point, my diet was basically devoid of nutrients (until the age of eighteen, the only vegetables I consumed were french fries and tomato sauce) and was chock-full of all the empty-calorie junk food my body didn't need.

Now I know with absolute confidence that the answer to "What are you eating?" will have a huge effect on one's overall health. But it wasn't a doctor or dermatologist—or even an adult, for that matter—who first asked me that question. In fact, it was a peer, someone my own age whom I met in college. She casually mentioned the acne I complained about may have been caused by what I was eating.

A novel idea, I thought. But I was desperate and willing to try anything. I bought a few books on the subject, and the rest is history. I cleared up my acne by changing my diet—something no pill, potion, or doctor had been able to do—lost twenty pounds (9 kg), and stopped getting sick as often as I used to. Soon, researching the food-health connection took over my life—and eventually shaped my career.

Before my food-changes-everything epiphany, I thought that food only affected body weight (which is why I'd peel the fried coating off my chicken nug-gets whenever I was on a "diet"). It never occurred to me there was a difference between "real food" and "edible food-like substances," as Michael Pollan dubbed them in his book *The Omnivore's Dilemma* (2006). These are items available in grocery stores that look like food, smell like food, and maybe even taste like food—but they come from a laboratory instead of a farm and provide little, if any, nutrition. And, in my opinion, that means they aren't really food.

I now know that what we eat affects everything from our skin's appearance to our immunity to our memory and learning ability to our cancer risk and so much more. It's taken me a while to get here, though.

I wrote *The Real Food Grocery Guide* to serve as the manual I wish I had when I was making the switch to real, nourishing foods that support health—the stuff our bodies were actually designed to eat in the first place.

As a certified integrative nutrition health coach, I've worked with hundreds of people, from young professionals and seasoned executives, to moms, celebs, and everyone in between. And I designed this book to provide practical, useful information that you, too, can easily apply to your own life—as soon as your next trip to the grocery store.

The principles contained in this book have dramatically changed my health and the health of my family, and I sincerely hope they'll do the same for you. May this book help you understand what you're eating and guide you to make healthier choices—for good.

With gratitude,
Maria

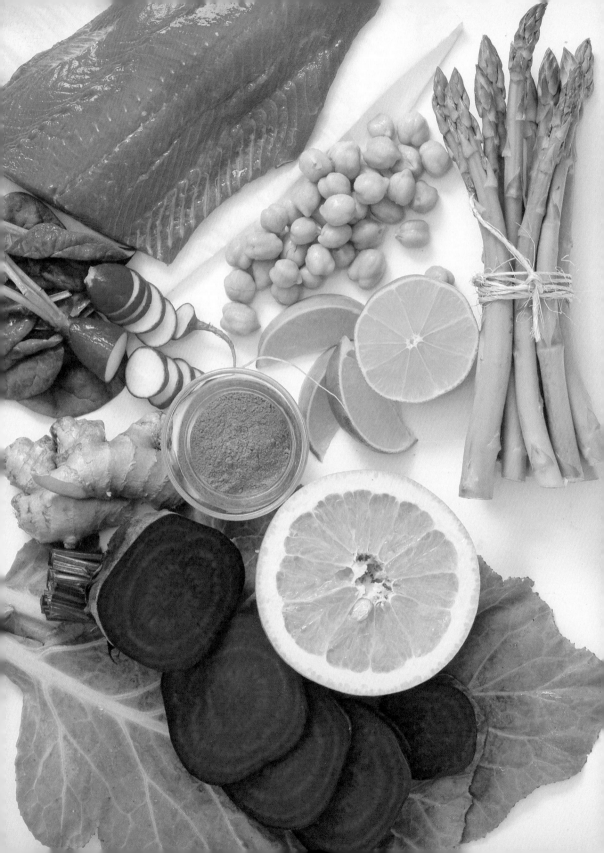

PART I

MAKING SMART CHOICES

A Return to Real Food. Food does much more than just satisfy our hunger. It provides the fuel our bodies need for thinking, moving, growing, repairing, and living. Our diet doesn't just affect weight: It also affects nearly every physical process, organ, function, and disease. As our current health and wellness statistics attest, our reliance on convenience foods instead of real foods has resulted in a health crisis of epic proportions. The good news, though, is that we can reverse weight gain and common ailments while moving toward optimum health by shifting to a real-food diet.

CHAPTER 1

THE CASE FOR EATING HOW NATURE INTENDED

"People *pay* you to take them around the grocery store?"

At first glance, the idea that you need a tour guide to navigate your local grocery store might sound odd. And you'd certainly be forgiven for thinking everything sold at a food store is actually *food*. But the fact is we're constantly bombarded with food-like impostors—especially as grocery stores continue to increase their square footage to cram in more items, while non-grocery retailers, such as drugstores and office supply stores, have added edible items to their offerings. These highly refined products do more to detract from our health than support it. And they're taking a toll on our health.

According to the Centers for Disease Control and Prevention (CDC), as of 2012, 69 percent of the U.S. population is overweight or obese, while one in two men and one in three women will get cancer at some point in their lifetimes. Though most people are well aware of the food-weight connection, the food-cancer connection is not as well publicized. The American Cancer Society has stated that at least one-third of all annual cancer deaths can be linked to poor diet, excess weight, and inactivity. That means that close to two hundred thousand lives annually could be saved by a real-food diet and an active lifestyle. Plus, some types of cancer have a much stronger connection to diet: for example, as much as 70 percent of colorectal cancer deaths may be diet related.

This means that it's now "normal" to be overweight, unhealthy, or both. So we need to ask ourselves another question. *Why?*

What Happened to Our Nutrition Education?

How did you learn what to eat and from whom? For many people, our parents shaped our eating habits. What you ate growing up probably isn't too far off from what you eat as an adult. But who taught *them* what to eat?

You might not realize it, but much of what you think you know about food and nutrition probably came from the food industry itself. You probably learned that milk supports bone health in the celebrity-studded *Got Milk?* ads sponsored by the American Dairy Association. You may have picked up the idea that fat-free or low-fat dairy products, such as yogurt or cheese, are healthier than full-fat versions from the very companies that produce them.

Or, you may have been convinced by a gyrating pop star in a dazzling TV commercial that a zero-calorie "diet" soda is better for your waistline than regular soda.

All of these ads and beliefs are false—and each is debunked in the chapters that follow—but the marketing campaigns surrounding them are quite memorable. These ads and others like them are a big part of what shapes our eating habits. But what about actual science or nutrition education?

Nutrition education in school is minimal, and what *is* taught can be downright misleading. Personally, I can't remember much in the way of nutrition instruction in school, but I do remember frequenting the chip- and cookie-filled vending machines that lined our hallways. In the cafeteria—aside from the occasional sad-looking apple—the only signs of fruit and vegetables were french fries and the tomato paste on pizza. (In hindsight, it's not terribly surprising, though, as the current U.S. Department of Agriculture [USDA] guidelines do qualify french fries and tomato paste on pizza as vegetable servings.)

My teachers may have glossed over the USDA food pyramid in a gym or health class, but I became much better acquainted with it at home. And I have General Mills to thank for that. Every morning I stared at a giant version of the pyramid plastered on the back of my Cheerios box as I shoveled spoonful after spoonful into my mouth: I'd eat as many as two or three bowls at a sitting, hurrying toward the six to eleven servings of "bread, cereal, rice, and pasta" it advised I eat each day. I thought there was a scientific reason for this. But just like the TV commercials and magazine ads, it, too, was propaganda.

The pyramid that shaped my early understanding of the ideal diet also shaped school and hospital food programs, not to mention dietitians' education and recommendations.

However—unbeknown to me—the pyramid was getting flak from scientists who felt it ignored the latest research and misled the public. This led to multiple iterations of the pyramid since its introduction in 1992. But some professionals in the nutrition and scientific communities have objected to it all along. Why? Because with each iteration it becomes more obvious that science is being replaced by economic interests.

In fact, after the most current version—the USDA's MyPlate—was released in June 2011, Harvard School of Public Health quickly published its own version, called the Healthy Eating Plate. On its website, the most prestigious research university in the country stated that it felt compelled to create unbiased nutrition guidelines "based exclusively on science and unsullied by political or commercial pressures from food industry lobbyists." Yikes. What's worse, though, is that the USDA's version is currently taught in schools and guides federal nutrition programs, including dietitian programs and school lunches.

As for doctors, often considered the gatekeepers of our health, they're hardly more educated about food and nutrition than the public. Growing up, my doctor's dietary advice was limited to chicken soup for colds and Gatorade for stomach flus to "replenish electrolytes." He didn't seem to mind that the sports drink contained sugar, artificial food colors linked to hyperactivity, or the synthetic chemical BVO that could build up in the body and become toxic. (BVO, short for brominated vegetable oil, was first marketed as a flame retardant and is banned from food use in Europe, India, and Japan. After strong consumer petitioning in 2014, BVO was removed from Gatorade, and parent company PepsiCo vowed to remove the ingredient from all its products—as did Coca-Cola—but at the time of writing it still remains in certain drinks.)

In my doctor's defense, though, I bet he was one of many pediatricians who received direct mail from Gatorade in the mid-1990s as part of its public relations campaign specifically targeting pediatricians. Due to his (likely) lack of nutrition training, he was probably completely unaware of the side effects of the ingredients: In fact, the average American doctor recieves fewer than twenty-four hours of nutrition instruction during his or her entire medical school education. The good news is that a small but growing number of doctors—particularly functional medicine practitioners—are incorporating real-food dietary recommendations into their practices after additional training or research.

Without a strong, unbiased education in nutrition, children, adults, and doctors alike are apt to be swayed by the pseudoscience the food industry pushes. And with an annual advertising spend of billions of dollars, it's nearly impossible to escape food industry advertising—no matter how hard you try.

The Gray Area of Food Marketing

When it comes to food advertising, the difference between reality and what's printed on the box is often a murky area. For example, in 2012, a series of lawsuits were brought against Tropicana for false advertising. Cartons of Tropicana claim the juice is "natural" and "100 percent orange juice." The lawsuits alleged that the juice undergoes heavy processing that's lengthy and complicated—a far cry from the famous image of an orange with a straw stuck into it that appears on the front of the package. In addition, after the oranges are squeezed, the juice is stored in giant holding tanks where it's stripped of its oxygen so it won't spoil while it sits there for months—or up to a year—before further

processing. Aromas, coloring, and flavor packs are then added to make it smell, look, and taste the same year-round. Tropicana doesn't list them in the ingredients list, however. What's the reasoning? They're derived from oranges. But after all the manipulation and chemical deconstruction used to make these ingredients, it's safe to say they no longer resemble anything found in nature.

At the time of writing, those suits are still open, but Tropicana's parent company, PepsiCo, settled another false advertising suit for its Naked Juice brand in 2013. At the time of the suit, labels on the product claimed it was "natural" and "non-GMO," but the bottles actually contained both synthetic and genetically modified (GMO) ingredients. GMO ingredients are discussed in chapter 12.

Because of the lax regulation of the food industry, there can be a great deal of difference between what you think you're getting and what you're actually getting when you purchase a food product. Worse, the industry doesn't only use poetic license when it comes to buzzwords such as "natural" or "non-GMO." Manufacturers often get in trouble for unsubstantiated health claims and deceptive marketing, too. Stories (and lawsuits) such as these abound.

PUSHING PSEUDOSCIENCE AS FACT
What's even more troubling are the ways in which the food industry uses its deep pockets to skew public opinion on serious health and food issues.

Take, for example, the idea that you can eat whatever you want as long as you exercise and still maintain a healthy weight. It's a commonly held belief, but it hasn't actually been proven. Still, it's repeated over and over again in the media. Parents and politicians complain that the lack of gym class is linked to the obesity epidemic; the most recent

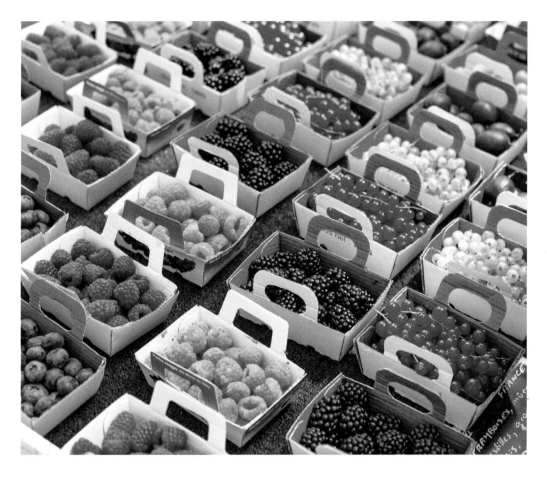

federal initiative to combat childhood obesity is called "Let's Move!" and fitness magazines often tout workouts for weight loss.

But numerous studies show that physical activity does not have a significant effect on weight. For example, a meta-analysis published in the *Journal of the Academy of Nutrition and Dietetics*, which included eight studies representing more than one thousand people, found that when a consistent diet was maintained, increasing workouts from less than one and one-half hours per week to three to five hours per week over the course of one full year led to an average weight loss of just three to four pounds (1.4 to 1.8 kg). You could healthfully lose that amount in as little

as two weeks by changing your diet. Another meta-analysis published in the journal *PLOS ONE* that examined the relationship between fat mass and physical activity in children found no association between the two and concluded that physical activity may not be the key determinant of unhealthy weight gain in children.

Now, there is no question that exercise is a critical part of a healthy lifestyle. It has many proven benefits: It supports the immune system, balances blood sugar, aids elimination, protects against heart disease and certain cancers, lowers stress levels, boosts mood, supports hormonal health, and may even prolong your life. But weight loss? Although

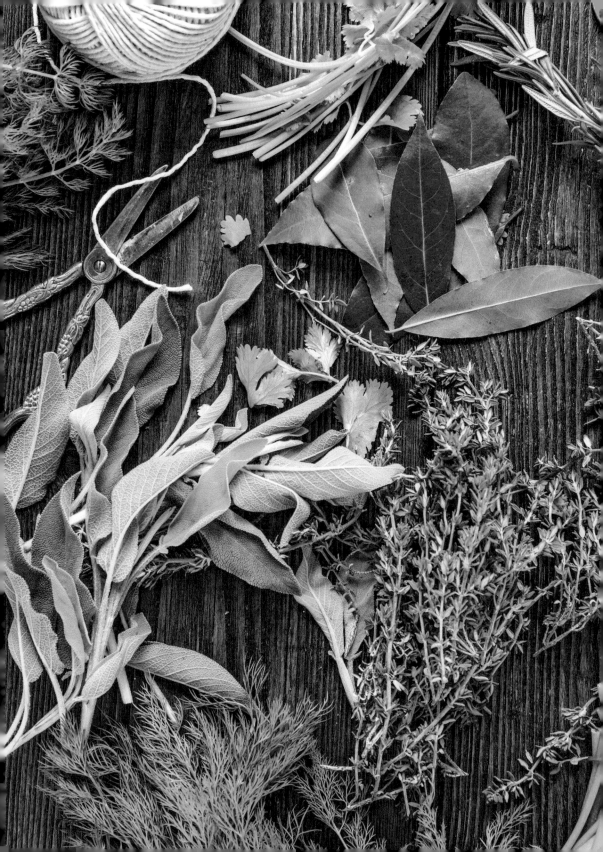

it certainly doesn't hurt—and can help, to a limited extent—science just doesn't show that it has as large an effect on the scale as the junk food industry would like you to believe. This myth is one perpetuated across the food industry.

For example, Coca-Cola has been caught spending millions of dollars funding a pseudoscience group to churn out studies that promote this misleading—even false—concept. In August 2015, Anahad O'Connor broke a story in the *New York Times*, reporting that the company helped bankroll a dubious organization called the Global Energy Balance Network, a nonprofit that claimed to research the causes of obesity but that was known primarily for promoting the idea that lack of exercise—not poor diet—was largely the cause of the obesity epidemic.

After Coca-Cola's $1.5 million donation was exposed, flak from consumer groups and scientists followed. Shortly afterward, in November 2015, the Global Energy Balance Network announced it would discontinue operations immediately. What the debacle brought to light, though, was that the food industry can, and does, pay scientists to conduct research that supports its bottom line—despite the actual health implications for the public. It can, and does, go so far as to obtain dubious research published in prestigious medical journals and promoted by researchers at conferences and through social media, which ultimately disseminates flawed science to the masses.

The idea of exercise as antidote for weight gain is so widespread now it's hard to escape. The truth is, you can work out like a maniac and still have trouble losing weight if you're not eating right. But the junk food industry, which has seen sales slip as Americans begin to turn away from it, is a multibillion dollar industry that won't go down without a fight.

IT'S NOT JUST THE FOOD GIANTS

Although it's not surprising that the food industry has its own self-interest in mind, it's disturbing that it has coaxed the country's nutrition professionals to collaborate with it. The Academy of Nutrition and Dietetics (AND) is the organization that accredits college and university educational programs for dietetics and grants certification to individuals as registered dietitians (RD) once they complete the nutrition requirements and pass the national certification exam. Registered dietitians have to complete seventy-five hours of continuing education units every five years to maintain their credential, which AND also oversees.

AND states it is committed to "improving the nation's health and advancing the profession of dietetics through research, education, and advocacy," but as a nonprofit that seeks corporate sponsorships, it doesn't appear to be immune to the food industry's whims. Corporate contributions are a significant source of income for AND, generating more than $1.1 million in 2015, about 5 percent of the total revenue for the Academy. The AND Foundation, which reports income separately and funds public education, scholarships, awards, and food and nutrition research, received about 51 percent of its revenue from corporate contributions.

Some of the most loyal and longstanding sponsors of AND include the National Dairy Council; ConAgra Foods (makers of Reddi-wip, Chef Boyardee, and Banquet frozen dinners); Kellogg's; and General Mills. In 2015, the top AND sponsors were the National Dairy Council and Abbott Nutrition (makers of Pedialyte and Similac), followed by Coca-Cola, General Mills, Kellogg's, McCormick, PepsiCo, and Unilever. Many of these companies have been involved with AND for more than a decade.

Plus when it comes to controversial health issues, AND typically takes a pro-industry stance. For example, when New York City was considering a ban on extra-large sodas, AND opposed it. It has also opposed a soda tax and GMO labeling. And it has approved continuing education courses sponsored by Coca-Cola, PepsiCo, Kraft Foods, and Nestlé for registered dietitians as part of their license requirements. You don't have to have a Ph.D. in nutrition to know these companies aren't exactly famous for their healthy fare—so why are they sponsoring nutrition classes and events for the professionals who are supposed to keep us healthy?

In a scathing exposé by lawyer and food activist Michele Simon, examples of messages taught in Coca-Cola–sponsored continuing education courses include the following: Sugar is not harmful to children; aspartame is completely safe; and the Institute of Medicine is too restrictive in its school nutrition standards. The Wheat Council has hosted classes that claim gluten intolerance is just a fad, not a real medical problem. The Corn Refiners Association has sponsored lectures that insist that high fructose corn syrup is no different than regular sugar and cannot be linked to the obesity epidemic—despite a growing body of evidence that suggests otherwise. And companies such as McDonald's have been known to sponsor and provide lunch for annual RD conferences. Though AND insists its classes and position on health issues are not influenced by its sponsors, it's hard not to see a connection here.

Although not well known outside the industry, these conflicts of interest have spurred much criticism among health advocates and nutrition professionals, including registered dietitians. Dietitians for Professional Integrity is a group that advocates for greater financial transparency and ethical sponsorships within the Academy of Nutrition and Dietetics and is vociferously opposed to sponsorship by corporate food giants such as Coca-Cola and PepsiCo. (In a win for public health, after the backlash Coca-Cola received for funding research to downplay the obesity epidemic, it didn't renew its AND sponsorship in 2016.)

The infiltration of the food industry into nutrition education and the deep food industry pockets that pay nutrition professionals to "consult" for or approve their products is a symbiotic relationship that ends up being detrimental to the health of our nation.

So, thanks to food industry advertising, misleading dietary recommendations, and the fact that the largest organization of nutritional professionals is in bed with major players in the food industry, much of what you think you know about food is probably wrong.

Calorie Schmalorie

Speaking of widespread misconceptions about food, the "calorie in, calorie out" theory for weight loss and health is probably one of the most established. Many, if not most, people who decide to embark on a weight-loss regimen begin to count calories to ensure they take in fewer calories than they burn. But the problem with the "you can eat whatever you want as long as you exercise it off" theory is that all calories *are not* created equal.

More and more research shows it's not only the *quantity*, but—more importantly—the *quality* of calories that counts when it comes to weight loss and overall health. In other words, you should be more concerned with the *ingredients* you're eating than the calorie count on the nutrition facts panel. A study by Harvard researchers published in the *Journal*

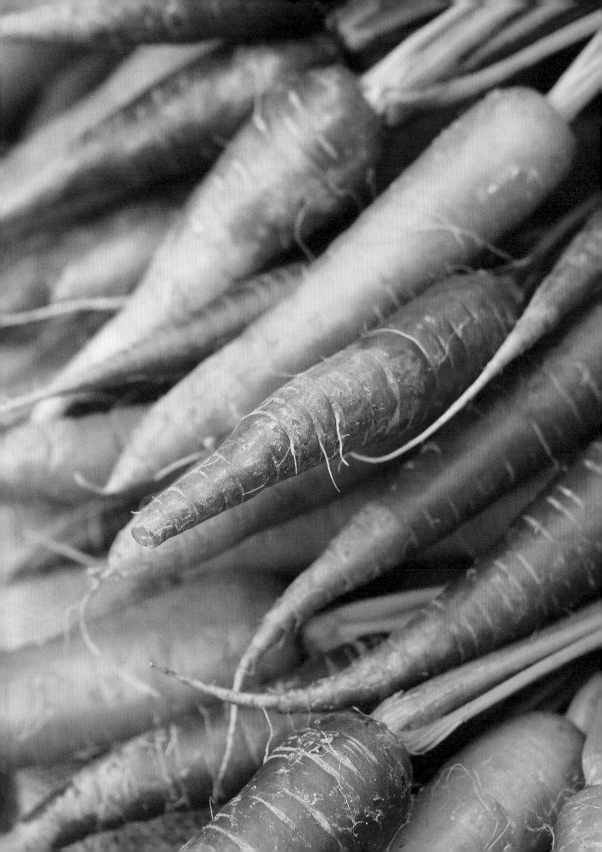

of the American Medical Association demonstrated that when calorie intakes were equal, diets made up of low-glycemic foods (those that have a minimal effect on blood sugar) led to the most desirable weight loss and health outcome. Low-glycemic foods are real foods. They include unrefined, minimally processed foods such as vegetables, fruit, whole grains, beans, nuts, fish, and chicken.

During the study, the authors monitored twenty-one overweight and obese participants over the course of six months. Participants were advised to follow either a low-fat diet, a low-glycemic diet, or a very low-carb diet. Those who followed the low-fat diet had the hardest time losing weight or keeping it off. The rate at which their bodies burned calories (known as energy expenditure) plummeted by as much as three hundred calories, which is the equivalent of one hour of moderately intense physical activity. This slower energy metabolism would likely lead to weight gain over time.

Those in the very low-carb camp experienced the highest energy expenditure, which suggests greater ease when it comes to burning calories and losing weight. But they experienced negative side effects too, such as elevated levels of the stress hormone cortisol and increased inflammation—which, in the long run, the study notes, may promote adiposity (fat gain), insulin resistance, and cardiovascular disease, as observed in epidemiological studies. Finally, the participants following the low-glycemic diet burned slightly fewer calories compared to the very low-carb diet, but without the negative side effects, so researchers deemed this diet the most desirable in terms of overall health outcomes.

Though this study is small, it challenges the age-old dietary dogma that a calorie is just a calorie. It demonstrates that when calorie counts are equal, the source of the calorie influences your metabolism and how easily you lose—or gain—weight.

Another, much larger study by Harvard researchers looked at the effects of dietary changes on weight and was able to pinpoint specific foods for their propensity to contribute either to weight gain or loss. Published in the *New England Journal of Medicine*, the study followed more than 120,000 healthy men and women over the course of twenty years. It discovered that the foods most strongly associated with weight gain were potato chips, potatoes, sugar-sweetened beverages, and both processed and unprocessed red meats. Foods shown to be associated with weight loss were vegetables, whole grains, fruits, nuts, and yogurt.

The findings suggest that choosing high-quality, unprocessed, mostly plant-based foods—also known as real foods—is an important factor in helping individuals lose weight (or maintain a healthy weight). This is likely because real food generally keeps blood sugar stable, regulates hunger, and keeps you satiated while delivering an abundance of nutrients through a low number of calories. Real foods take up stomach space, so to speak, and crowd out other less healthy options, such as processed foods and red meat, which tend to be low in nutrients and high in calories.

What Is Real Food?

Real food is what you find around the periphery of the grocery store. It's all the edible products Mother Nature gave us, in their unadulterated forms: fresh vegetables, fruit, whole grains, legumes, nuts, seeds, eggs, fish, and unprocessed meat.

So, what does that make everything else—like the brightly colored packages that fill up the center of the supermarket, or the processed and novel meat products, or the baked goods with a nearly immortal shelf life? Journalist and author Michael Pollan has dubbed them "edible food-like substances," but others use the more affectionate term "Frankenfoods." They look like food, smell like food, and taste like food, but they bear no more resemblance to actual food than the plastic stuff a seven-year-old would serve you at a tea party.

Highly refined foods such as these are associated with a range of ills, from weight gain to heart disease to cancer. These substances don't support our health and, in my opinion, don't qualify as real food. Now, this doesn't mean you can never eat anything out of a package again, nor does it mean that everything in a package is necessarily bad. But because these food imposters are so prevalent, it's helpful to have a tour guide take you through the modern grocery store to point you in the right direction. After all, food affects your entire physical and mental well-being, not just your waistline.

Hundreds, if not thousands, of ailments—from acne and migraines to mental fog and

Real Food [reel food]; noun

1. Any nourishing substance that originates from Mother Nature—not a factory—and is consumed to promote health, provide energy, and sustain life.

2. Fresh vegetables, fruit, whole grains, legumes, nuts, seeds, and, optionally, organic eggs, wild fish, and unprocessed meat.

digestive issues—can be addressed with food. In the chapters to come, you'll learn how food can improve everything from your waistline to your complexion, from your athletic performance to your IQ, and even influence your cancer risk.

THE FOOD & HEALTH CONNECTION

Remember that friend in high school? The one who could eat anything—hamburgers, fries, mac and cheese—and never gain an ounce? Meanwhile, you put on weight by just looking at those foods. It didn't seem fair.

Well, don't be too jealous. Food affects people differently. But make no mistake: It *does* affect each of us. Some people may gain weight from junk food, others may suffer from skin breakouts, stomachaches, migraines, high cholesterol—or even end up with more serious diseases. In fact, about half of all American adults—117 million individuals—have one or more preventable chronic diseases, many of which are related to poor-quality eating patterns and physical inactivity. As you'll see following, six of the eight leading causes of death in the United States are diet- or lifestyle-related. (The other two are due to accidents.)

Internationally, the statistics in high-income countries, including but not limited to England, Australia, and New Zealand, are similar. Noncommunicable diseases accounted for 68 percent of global deaths in 2012, with cardiovascular diseases, cancers, diabetes, and chronic lung diseases being the most prevalent. Cardiovascular diseases took 17.5 million lives that year and were responsible for three of every ten deaths.

Even though we consume it every day, many of us have no clue how food *really* affects our individual bodies. Many people are unaware it could be the culprit behind breakouts, migraines, mood swings, digestive troubles, lack of energy, memory issues, learning impairment, decreased immunity, and even an increased cancer risk. The truth is, though, that food can be our most powerful medicine—or our most toxic poison.

To understand how, let's use a car as a metaphor. If you fill your car with fuel—either premium or regular—your car will run. But the car with the higher-quality premium fuel will, generally, outperform its lower-quality counterpart. It's the same with food. Yes, your body will still function on a diet of low-quality junk food, but how will you feel? How will you look? How will your body perform? Probably not at its peak.

Countless studies connect food with health and suggest that you really *are* what you eat. This chapter outlines the dietary links to two of the leading causes of death (heart disease and cancer), plus a host of other less serious but common ailments, further supporting the case for switching to real food.

How Food Affects Heart Health

Heart disease is the number one cause of death globally, but it doesn't have to be this way. Changing our diets and lifestyles—factors over which we have complete control—can go a long way toward reducing the risk of heart disease. In fact, the American Heart Association expresses this quite clearly on its website: "Your lifestyle is not only your best defense against heart disease and stroke, it's also your responsibility." The website also lists the lifestyle factors that can mitigate your risk, including quitting smoking; being physically active every day; maintaining a healthy weight; reducing stress; limiting alcohol; and enjoying a proper diet, noting that, "a healthy diet is one of the best weapons you have to fight cardiovascular disease."

The association's recommendations, no doubt, have been at least partly influenced by the work of top cardiologist and researcher Dean Ornish, M.D., who was the first to show clinically that heart disease can be reversed through specific diet and lifestyle changes. Through a combination of a whole-food, plant-based diet, stress management, physical activity, and the creation of a support network, he has helped thousands of patients not only halt heart disease, but reverse it, too. In one early study, forty-eight patients with moderate to severe coronary heart disease were divided into two groups: one that followed the intensive lifestyle changes mentioned or one that received only the care normally provided in the Western medical system.

The participants who made the diet and lifestyle changes saw a decrease in plaque buildup in their coronary arteries (a 4.5 percent improvement after one year and a 7.9 percent improvement after five years), whereas the control group that didn't make the changes saw an increase in the narrowing of their coronary arteries (a 5.4 percent worsening after one year and a 27.7 percent worsening after five years).

How Food Affects Cancer

No one wants to hear his or her doctor mutter the C-word, but as mentioned previously, statistics suggest one in two men and one in three women in the United States will be diagnosed with cancer during their lifetime. That places the United States in sixth place for highest cancer incidences globally, preceded by Denmark, France, Australia, Belgium, and Norway, according to World Cancer Research Fund International. The United Kingdom ranks twenty-second. A University of Texas study suggests that as many as 90 to 95 percent of cancer incidences are related to environment and lifestyle factors, including cigarette smoking; diet (particuarly those rich in fried foods and red meat); excessive alcohol consumption; sun exposure; environmental pollutants; infections; stress; obesity; and physical inactivity. "Of all cancer-related deaths, almost 25 to 30 percent are due to tobacco; as many as 30 to 35 percent are linked to diet; [and] about 15 to 20 percent are due to infections," said the authors. Other studies have shown similar results. One study published in the journal *Nature* suggested that 70 to 90 percent of cancer cases could be attributed to outside, environmental factors, while less than 10 to 30 percent could be linked to intrinsic, or genetic, factors.

No single food or nutrient alone can protect you from cancer because everything you ingest works together synergistically. But research suggests that, overall, a real food or whole food, plant-based diet can help lower the risk for certain types of cancer. Foods that demonstrate the most promising potential to lower cancer risk include cruciferous

FACT Top Eight Causes of Death in the United States per Year

Cause of Death	Number of Deaths
Heart disease	611,105
Cancer	584,881
Iatrogenic	180,000*
Chronic lower respiratory diseases	149,205
Accidents (unintentional injuries)	130,557
Stroke (cerebrovascular diseases)	128,978
Alzheimer's disease	84,767
Diabetes	75,578

Source: Centers for Disease Control and Prevention Deaths: *Final Data for 2013*.

*An iatrogenic death is unintentionally caused by a physician, surgeon, medical treatment, or diagnostic procedure. However, a study led by Barbara Starfield, M.D., and published in the *Journal of the American Medical Association* indicates that number may be much higher, as many as 284,000.

FACT Top Seven Causes of Death in the World

Cause of Death	Number of Deaths
Ischemic heart disease	7.4 million
Stroke	6.7 million
Trachea, bronchus, lung cancers	1.6 million
Chronic obstructive pulmonary disease (COPD)	3.1 million
Lower respiratory infections	3.1 million
Diabetes mellitus	1.5 million
Hypertensive heart disease	1.1 million

Source: World Health Organization, 2012.

vegetables (cabbage, broccoli, and cauliflower), legumes (beans, peas, and lentils), and alliums (onions and garlic). They are discussed in detail in chapters 4 and 6.

How Food Affects Brain Health, Memory & Learning Ability

Fernando Gomez-Pinilla, Ph.D., a UCLA professor of neurosurgery and physiological science, has spent years studying the effects of food, exercise, and sleep on the brain. "Food is like a pharmaceutical compound that affects the brain," he says. "Diet, exercise, and sleep have the potential to alter our brain health and mental function. This raises the exciting possibility that changes in diet are a viable strategy for enhancing cognitive abilities, protecting the brain from damage, and counteracting the effects of aging." One dietary change that can have a positive effect on brain health is adding more omega-3–rich foods—not supplements—to your diet. Omega-3 fatty acids are found in wild salmon, mackerel, and walnuts and have been shown to improve learning and memory—and may even provide protection against certain psychological disorders, including depression, schizophrenia, and dementia.

Although you may already be aware of of omega-3's brain benefits, beware that the wildly promoted omega-3 and fish oil *supplements* may not provide them. A study published in the *Journal of the American Medical Association*, one of the largest and lengthiest of its kind, found that taking omega-3 supplements over the course of five years did *not* slow cognitive decline among four thousand participants. So, instead of relying on supplements, eat the real foods that contain them, and do so regularly.

Blueberries are also noted for their brain-boosting benefits. In a Harvard study published in the *Annals of Neurology*, researchers followed sixteen thousand women, most in their seventies, over six years and found that those with the highest intake of blueberries delayed their memory decline by as many as two and a half years.

And just as certain foods support brain health, others may diminish it. Moms have always known that sugar can cause kids to "bounce off the walls," becoming hyperactive and inattentive, and it may make your thinking a little foggy, too. A small study published in *Neurology* found that higher blood sugar levels in people were associated with a decline in memory. Multiple animal studies have yielded similar results, with high sugar intake impairing both long- and short-term memory. Though these studies are small and further research needs to be done, simply observing how you feel or think after consuming large amounts of sugar can tell you a great deal about how your body reacts to it.

How Food Affects Digestive Health

This one isn't as intuitive as it sounds. Chronic constipation, gas, bloating, and diarrhea are common, but precisely because they're so common, many of us tend to shrug them off as "normal" without realizing our favorite foods may be to blame.

I've had many clients come to me for help with weight loss and at the first session, assure me they had no digestive issues. But upon further prodding, they'd admit they were always gassy or bloated or hadn't had a bowel movement in three days. When I'd ask why they didn't tell me that right off the bat, most clients responded, "I thought that was normal." Yes, a little gas here and there is normal, but being mistaken for a pregnant woman when your tummy balloons with gas after a meal or considering a successful

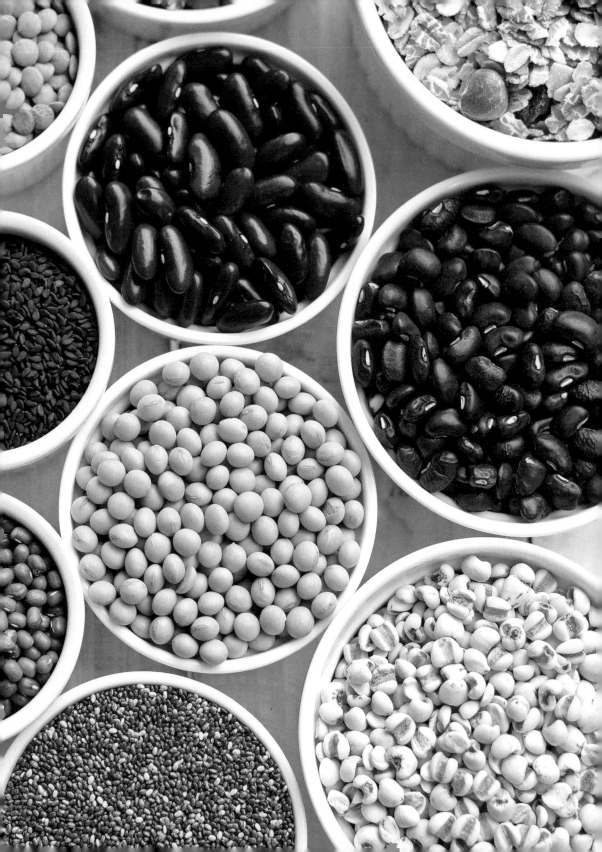

bowel movement to be a rare accomplishment is not. Though there are many possible causes for digestive distress, what we eat naturally plays a large role: After all, the food we ingest comes in direct contact with our digestive systems.

The Western medical establishment defines constipation as having bowel movements fewer than three times a week. In Eastern medical systems—including traditional Chinese medicine and Ayurveda (traditional Indian medicine designed to bring the mind and body into balance for overall healing)—anything less than one movement daily is cause for concern. I agree with the Eastern medicine perspective: If you eat every day, you should excrete every day. Plus, if you eat the recommended amounts of fruit, vegetables, legumes, and whole grains, it's unlikely you'll be going less than once per day.

If your pipes are backed up, it's probably a sign that your diet lacks adequate fiber-rich foods or water, although other factors—lack of exercise, magnesium, or fat; an unbalanced gut microbiome; or stress—can also be contributors. If the problem stems from a lack of fiber, include more fiber-rich foods and water in your diet. Taking a fiber supplement won't cut it because you miss out on all the other benefits of naturally fiber-rich foods. The reality is that at about three grams of fiber per teaspoon, you'd have to sprinkle on quite a few teaspoons to get within the recommended daily range. But when you start eating more plant-based real foods, your body will naturally move toward daily elimination.

The Best Diet for Health

In short, it's up to you to take control of your health, and you can start by taking control of what you eat. Study after study suggests that a whole food, plant-based diet free from refined and heavily processed foods is the ideal diet for health.

A healthy diet or lifestyle won't make you bulletproof to illness, but it can significantly lower your risk of developing one. When it comes to food, every morsel you put in your mouth becomes a building block for your blood, your cells, your organs, and your skin—so choose wisely. The rest of this book shows you how to do just that.

CHAPTER 3

REAL FOOD, REAL AFFORDABLE

"Healthy food is just too expensive."

If you've ever found yourself uttering those words, you're not alone. But, by now, you're probably beginning to realize that feeling good, looking your best, and being vibrantly healthy are invaluable. Still, an empty bank account certainly won't help your stress levels. So now that you understand why switching to real food is a wise choice for your health, this chapter shows you how to do it without emptying your wallet in the process.

It's All in Your Head . . .

When you take into account the real cost of cheap food (excess weight, low energy, diminished health, and chronic illness, plus all the diet programs, medications, and doctor appointments that accompany them), you may not be spending much money on food, but you're probably spending it elsewhere (Spanx, anyone?). When you think big picture and put it all into perspective, the health benefits afforded by eating real food justify the monetary cost in the long run.

. . . and May Not Be that Expensive After All

How true is it that real food is significantly more expensive? At first glance, an eight-ounce (225 g) bag of chips, which has nine servings and only costs $2 or $3, may seem like a bargain. The reality is, though, it's not unfathomable for one person to polish off an entire bag in one or two sittings. And it's also possible that same person could be hungry just a couple hours later. Empty-calorie processed foods may be cheap, but they are largely devoid of the fiber and nutrients that trigger satiety, resulting in the desire to consume more.

On the other hand, take cauliflower—a real food with plenty of health benefits. There may be some initial sticker shock at a price of $5, sure, but one large head—probably about three pounds (1.4 kg)—would easily serve four with a generous two-cup (200 g) portion. And if you've ever had two cups (200 g) of cauliflower, you know you're unlikely to be rummaging around the kitchen again soon afterward.

If you choose the right foods and shop at the right places, real food—particularly vegetables, fruit, beans, and legumes—can be affordable for everyone. The things truly on the more expensive side in natural food stores are the packaged products, such as dehydrated kale chips (which you really don't need) and meat (which, as you'll learn in chapter 8, is worth the added cost).

Where to Shop

Today, it's becoming increasingly easier and more affordable to access healthy food no matter where you live, thanks to the internet. In fact, you can eat healthfully without ever having to leave your house if you don't want to—and I'm not talking about takeout. Even if you live across the street from a health food store, ordering, at the very least, all your dry goods online can save both money and time. And, if you like, you can even order fresh organic produce and high-quality organic meat online as well.

But if you're a serious foodie like me and you love the ritual of shopping, nothing beats a walk through the grocery aisles or farmers' market stands where you can touch (and maybe taste) before you buy.

The pages that follow have resources to help you find farmers' markets, health food stores, and grocery stores, no matter where you live. And, if you love to cook, seriously consider joining a CSA (community supported agriculture) program. Your grocery shopping options, both in person and online, follow.

Remember, healthy eating is not just for health nuts, hippies, or the 1 percent. It's the right of every single person to have access to fresh, nourishing, delicious, affordable, and healthy food.

NATURAL GROCERS & HEALTH FOOD STORES

Mom-and-pop health food stores are one of my favorite places to shop because I know they carry what I like, and it allows me to support a fellow local business and health crusader, too. They typically have an edited assortment of goods, which excludes some of the conventional junk food more common in mainstream grocers and a wider variety of foods made more naturally. Remember, not everything sold in a *health* food store is necessarily *healthy* (vegan cookies, I'm looking at you).

Although health food stores were once the only places to carry organic produce, gluten-free crackers, and the like, more and more mainstream grocers and national chains are beginning to offer a decent and growing assortment of healthier options.

Most grocery stores are regional, so your best bet is to shop around your neighborhood to discover which grocer has the best assortment and prices.

Find a Natural Grocer or Health Food Store in Your Area

Aside from doing a Google search for "health food store in (your area)," check out www.organicstorelocator.com or www.happycow.net.

Maria's Favorite Natural Grocers

Northeast	South	Midwest	West	Nationwide	International
A Matter of Health, New York	Rainbow Blossom, Kentucky	Mariano's, Illinois	Rainbow Grocery, San Francisco	Whole Foods Market	Whole Foods Market, U.K.
Westerly Natural Market, New York	MOM's Organic Market, Maryland, Washington D.C.	Natural Grocers	Berkley Bowl, Berkley, California		Planet Organic, U.K.
Fairway Market, New York			Erewhon, Los Angeles, Calabasas, and Venice, California		Bio c' Bon, France
MOM's Organic Market, New Jersey. Pennsylvania, Virginia			Lassens Natural Foods & Vitamins, California		
			Mother's Market & Kitchen, California		
			New Seasons Market, Oregon, Washington, Northern California		

Maria's Favorite Natural Grocers
Above is a list of some of my favorite natural grocers across the globe. I hope you find one (or two) that become favorites, too.

NATIONAL CHAINS WITH HEALTHY & ORGANIC CHOICES

While the big national chains have not traditionally been the best places to find healthy options and top-quality organic produce, times are changing. Many major national chains have responded to consumer demand and now stock a variety of organic and healthy items.

Whole Foods Market
Whole Foods Market is a pioneer in the healthy grocery store space and has helped

make organic and natural foods more mainstream. It's an international chain with locations all over the United States, Canada, and the United Kingdom, offering a large assortment of organic produce and meat as well as high-quality packaged products.

Due to some higher price points in comparison to traditional grocers, Whole Foods Market has earned the nickname "whole paycheck"—but that's not entirely fair. The truth is you can find lots of bargains at Whole Foods. There are great sales; its private-label "365 Everyday Value" brand is economically priced; and it's hard to beat the assortment of healthy goods. If there's a Whole Foods Market near you, stretch your dollar by purchasing mostly fresh products, such as produce or meat, there and ordering nonperishables online through one of the following resources, where you'll find more competitively priced items because they don't have the overhead costs of a storefront.

Trader Joe's
Trader Joe's is a national chain known for being incredibly affordable. It has a large variety of organic offerings, although it has recently come under fire for being secretive about its supplier sources and for not having third-party verification to back up its claims that it is a non-GMO store.

💰 Money-Saving Tip

To keep grocery expenses down, shop from the weekly sales flyer, buy from the bulk section, and stick to fresh instead of packaged products as much as possible. Consider choosing store brands, which offer similar products at a more economical price than brand names.

❗ Expert Tip

When to Shop the Grocery Store

If you hate playing bumper shopping carts or waiting in checkout lines, avoid the grocery store at peak times and opt to go when they tend to be emptier.

Best times to hit the grocery store:

- Weeknights: 8 p.m. to 10 p.m.
- Weekends: 8 a.m. to 11 a.m.

Worst times to hit the grocery store:

- Weeknights: 5 p.m. to 8 p.m.
- Weekends: 12 p.ma. to 5 p.m.

Best time to shop online:

- Any time!

Because it does make organic foods so much more affordable than other grocery stores, I still think it's a great place to shop. But because it doesn't provide third-party verification of its non-GMO claims, if you're serious about avoiding GMOs (see chapter 12), I'd advise that you avoid products containing ingredients that are typically genetically modified, such as corn, canola, or soy—unless they are certified organic.

Walmart, Costco & Safeway
Large national chains, including Walmart, Costco, and Safeway, now stock a decent assortment of organic produce and healthier packaged products at excellent prices. Don't overlook these stores as an option. Costco stores exist all over the world, including Canada, Mexico, and Australia. In Europe, Walmart operates as Asda.

Find a Farmers' Market in Your Area

Use this site to find a farmers' market near you: www.localharvest.org/farmers-markets/.

Find a Food Co-op in Your Area

Aside from doing a Google search for "food co-op near (your city and state)," check out www.coopdirectory.org.

FARMERS' MARKETS

Most cities and towns offer a local farmers' market at least once a week, and I highly recommend you make it part of your weekly shopping if you can. Farm-fresh produce is bursting with flavor (and nutrients)—much more so than typical grocery store fare. In addition to local produce, you can usually find farm-fresh eggs, dairy, meat, fish, and, sometimes, prepared foods.

Organic produce is typically plentiful, although not all farms will be certified organic, which is a lengthy and expensive process. You may see farms that advertise as "no spray" or "no pesticide and herbicide," which should signal their products are grown with organic methods and are still an excellent choice. When in doubt, ask the farmer.

Although farmers' markets might not stock everything you need, they're a wonderful place to get your perishable ingredients for the week. By shopping at farmers' markets, you get better-tasting and more nutritious foods plus access to a wider variety of produce. You also support local farmers and the local economy by shopping at farmers' markets. You even help protect the environment by cutting down on pollution from shipping, packing materials, and conventional agriculture practices. Consider making it a Saturday or Sunday morning ritual with your family (or just time for yourself!).

Depending on where you live, farmers' markets will either be much cheaper than, on par with, or slightly more expensive than the grocery store. As for the pricier items, the flavor, freshness, and superior nutrition will usually more than make up for it. Don't be afraid to ask the farmer for a taste before you purchase something: They're usually happy to oblige. The first time you taste a freshly picked strawberry, you'll understand why I'm urging you to go!

FOOD CO-OPS

Food co-ops are cooperatively owned grocery stores in which you volunteer a few hours of your time to work at the store each month in exchange for access to high-quality—but low-priced—healthy foods all year long. You can expect to work one day or a few hours a month for groceries that are about 20 to 40 percent off retail price. If your average grocery bill is $100 a week, that's an approximate savings of between $1,000 and $2,000 a year.

More and more co-ops are springing up around the country, thanks to an increased awareness of healthy foods and the desire to make them affordable for all. If there's no co-op near you and you're feeling ambitious, why not start your own?

COMMUNITY SUPPORTED AGRICULTURE (CSA)

Community Supported Agriculture, or CSA, allows you to "buy a share" in a farm's output for a season. Each week, a local farmer will fill a box with perfectly ripe, in-season produce and deliver it to your home or a local pickup point. CSAs offer access to an abundance of

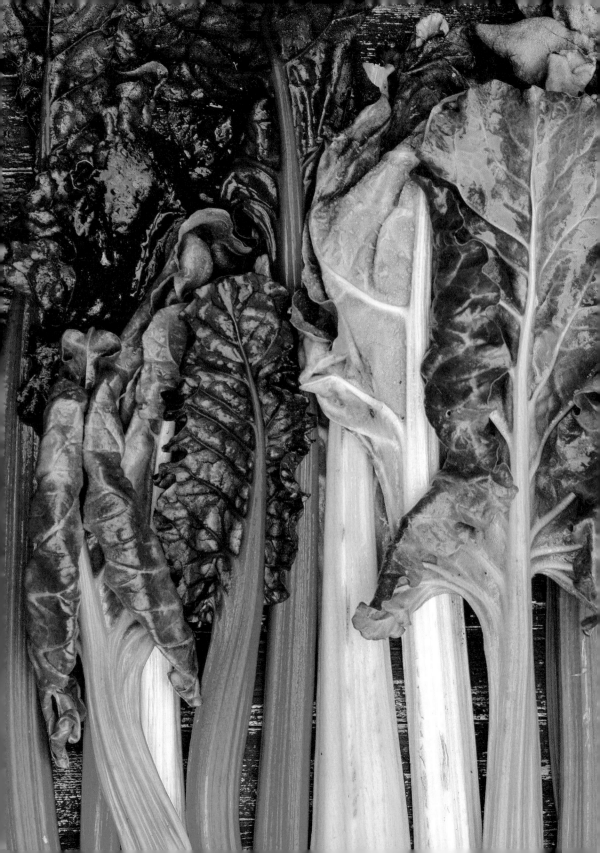

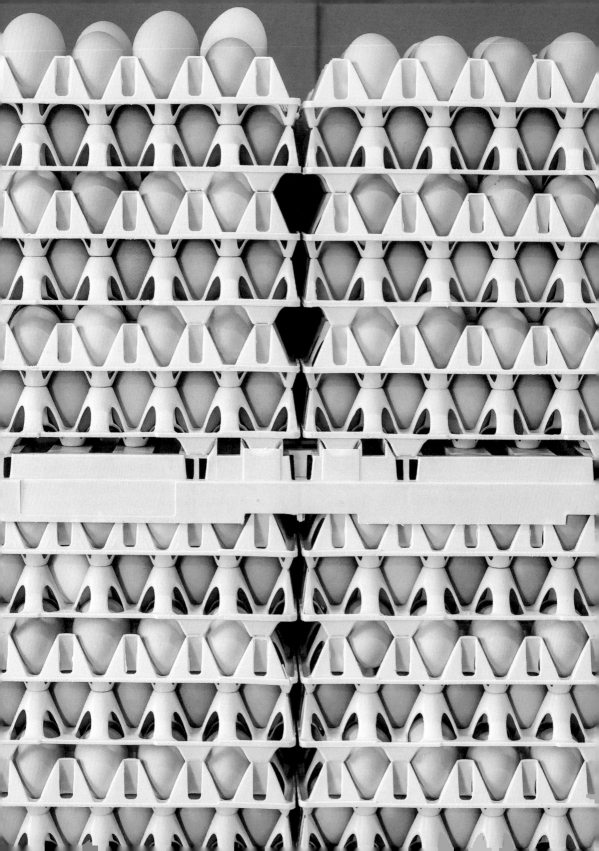

Find a CSA in Your Area

Locate a CSA in your area with this site: www.localharvest.org/csa/.

farm-fresh produce at a fraction of what you'd pay at the grocery store. Each CSA offers a different variety of goods, so research your options before choosing one. It's a great option if you're feeding a family or if you simply love to cook.

ONLINE

If you don't live near a health food store or have little to no time to grocery shop, these resources will afford you access to the healthiest foods, often at the lowest possible prices. In fact, it may make sense for everyone to shop online to save both time and money.

For pantry staples and packaged goods, check out the following resources.

- **Thrive Market, www.thrivemarket.com.** If Amazon, Whole Foods Market, and Costco had a baby, Thrive Market would be it. For a yearly membership fee (currently less than $5 per month), you get access to thousands of organic and healthy packaged products, including food, supplements, and beauty products—all at wholesale prices of 25 to 50 percent off, which more than justifies the membership fee. After personally using it and saving more than $1,000 in annual grocery costs, I'm happy to partner with Thrive Market. For a thirty-day free trial, go to www.thrivemarket.com/mm.

☯ Money-Saving Tip

To keep your dry bulk goods fresher longer, purchase large wide-mouth glass Mason jars with an airtight seal and a wide-mouth funnel. Transfer bulk goods into the jars when you get home. Though they're pretty, don't be tempted to store them in well-lit places such as the kitchen counter: Keep them away from sunlight, ideally in a closet or cupboard, to keep their contents fresh.

- **Vitacost, www.vitacost.com.** Vitacost stocks thousands of brand-name food items, supplements, and natural beauty items at up to 30 percent off grocery store prices. This is an excellent resource for dry and packaged goods: They have one of the widest assortments around.

- **Nuts.com, www.nuts.com.** Nuts.com offers a large variety of organic and conventional dry bulk goods, including nuts, seeds, dry beans, grains, and flours. The quality is excellent and orders arrive incredibly fast.

- **Eat Wild, www.eatwild.com.** This website offers a robust directory of local farms by state that provide fresh animal products, including organic meat, eggs, and dairy.

- **Instacart, www.instacart.com.** Instead of having its own warehouse or supply chain like the other resources in this list, for a small fee, Instacart sends a personal shopper to the local grocery store of your choice to pick up the exact items you select—no need to leave your house. Talk about convenience! Instacart serves most major cities.

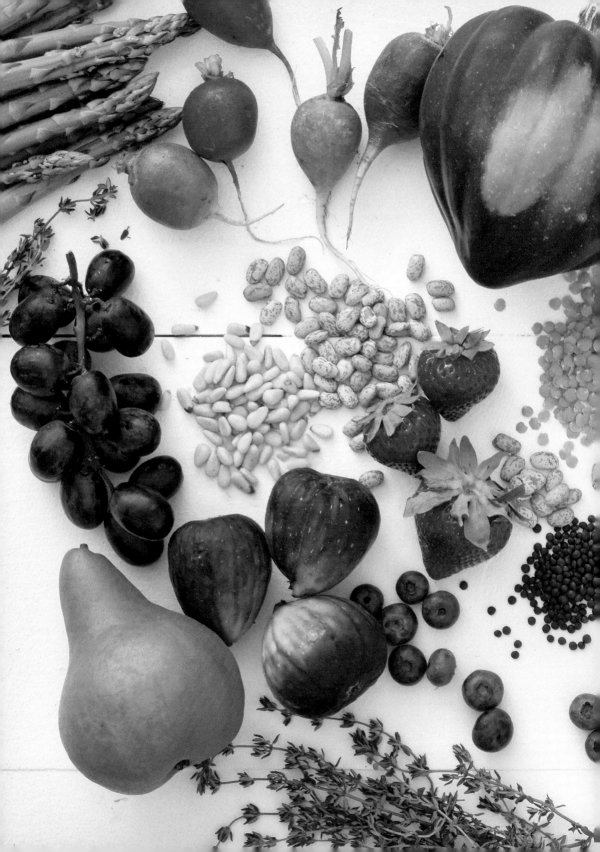

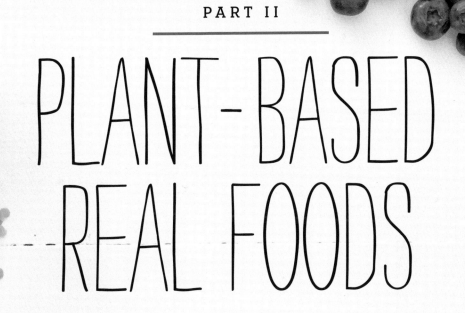

PART II

PLANT-BASED REAL FOODS

Selecting the Freshest & Most Nutritious Options. Plant-based whole foods are real foods at their finest. They're everything that comes from Mother Nature's bounty: vegetables, fruit, grains, legumes, beans, nuts, and seeds.

This section teaches you practically everything you need to know about plant-based real foods, including what their colors indicate, why it's important to "eat the rainbow," and why choosing local and organic is preferable, but not a deal breaker. It explores the health benefits and concerns of each food group and shows you how to select and store more than fifty of the most common fruits and vegetables so you'll never waste money on brown avocados or tasteless melons again.

CHAPTER 4

PRODUCE

Stacked high with fresh fruit and vegetables in a rainbow of colors, the produce section is the grocery store's most dazzling space. In metropolitan cities and specialty grocers, it sometimes includes exotic produce from far-off lands—but in terms of nutrition, the more "humble" fruits and veggies, such as apples, carrots, broccoli, and beets, are actually the stars of the show.

As you'll learn in this chapter, vegetables and fruit are some of the most nutritionally dense and health-promoting foods available to us. Many nutrition experts agree that for optimum health at least 50 percent of your plate should be comprised of vegetables or fruit at every meal. So, spend some time getting acquainted with this section because the bulk of what you buy should come from the produce aisles.

And, if you think you don't like vegetables or fruit, this section could change your mind—so don't skip it. I encourage you to sample new varieties or to retry the ones you think you don't like with different recipes, spices, and cooking techniques or, simply, a different cut of meat. Remember, when it comes to food, spices and texture change a lot! Think of overcooked, pale green, mushy broccoli versus crisp, lightly steamed, bright green broccoli: It's the same food, but the taste is worlds apart.

Produce Buzzwords

Make sure you know what you're buying. Learn the meaning behind these common terms to make the best choices in the produce section.

ORGANIC

Organic produce is grown without the use of toxic or persistent pesticides, synthetic fertilizers, sewage sludge, or irradiation. They are never GMO (genetically modified). They're a smart choice for many reasons. They are typically more nutritious; they're easier on the environment; and they help you avoid the toxic chemicals commonly used in conventional farming. Many common agricultural chemicals have been linked to serious health concerns, from brain damage to infertility to endocrine complications and even cancer.

> **FACT** **Organic versus Local**
>
> From a health standpoint, when purchasing any of the Dirty Dozen foods (see page 47), it's generally better to buy organic than local to avoid toxic agricultural chemicals. For the Clean Fifteen foods (see page 47) and most other produce, your exposure to chemicals is limited, so you may prefer buying local: It will probably taste better because it's likely to be fresher.

LOCAL

Local foods are grown or raised within a small geographic radius, typically within 50 to 150 miles (80 to 241 km) of wherever you purchase them. Because local foods are picked when ripe, travel shorter distances, and are sold more quickly, they're usually fresher. Fresher produce not only tastes better, it's also typically more nutritious. Local food protects the environment by cutting down on carbon dioxide emissions during shipping and also strengthens your local economy. When you buy farm-fresh, locally grown produce, you can rest assured it's seasonal. Beyond personal reasons, buying local is better for the environment and the local economy. If you're lucky, you'll be able to find local food that's also organic.

GENETICALLY MODIFIED (GMO)

Genetically modified fruits and vegetables have had their DNA altered. (Find out more about the concerns associated with GMO foods in chapter 12.) In the produce aisles, genetically modified foods include corn, papaya, zucchini, and yellow summer squash, although GMO apples and potatoes were recently approved and will soon make their way into grocery stores. Because GMO crops are so widespread, you can assume any of these foods in their conventional forms are GMO. If you'd like to enjoy non-GMO versions of these foods, always buy them organic.

Shared Benefits of Produce

Fruit and vegetables share many health benefits, so we'll discuss them in general before looking at each more specifically.

VITAMINS, MINERALS, ANTIOXIDANTS & PHYTOCHEMICALS

Fruit and vegetables are nature's multivitamins. They're packed with a wide variety of nutrients and phytochemicals that our bodies need to stay strong and healthy. The color of produce can be an indicator of which phytochemicals and antioxidants it contains, which is why it's important to include the entire rainbow of colors in your diet. Generally, the darker the hue, the more antioxidants it contains. So, eating plant-based foods in a variety of colors—especially rich, deep, dark hues—is an easy way to ensure you're getting the full spectrum of phytochemicals and nutrients to support vibrant health, without the need for a multivitamin supplement.

ANTI-INFLAMMATORY

More and more scientific research cites chronic inflammation as the root cause of many types of disease, including heart disease, Alzheimer's, and certain cancers. Vegetables and fruit fight inflammation in the body, protecting your overall health and offering some relief from the symptoms of inflammatory conditions, such as arthritis or fibromyalgia.

SATIETY

A wonderful attribute of many plant-based real foods, including vegetables and fruit, is their built-in portion control. Think of it this way: While it's incredibly easy to eat five (or fifteen!) cookies in one sitting, you're probably never going to sit down and eat five apples all at once. When you eat real foods loaded with fiber, your body knows when to stop, and you'll feel satiated longer.

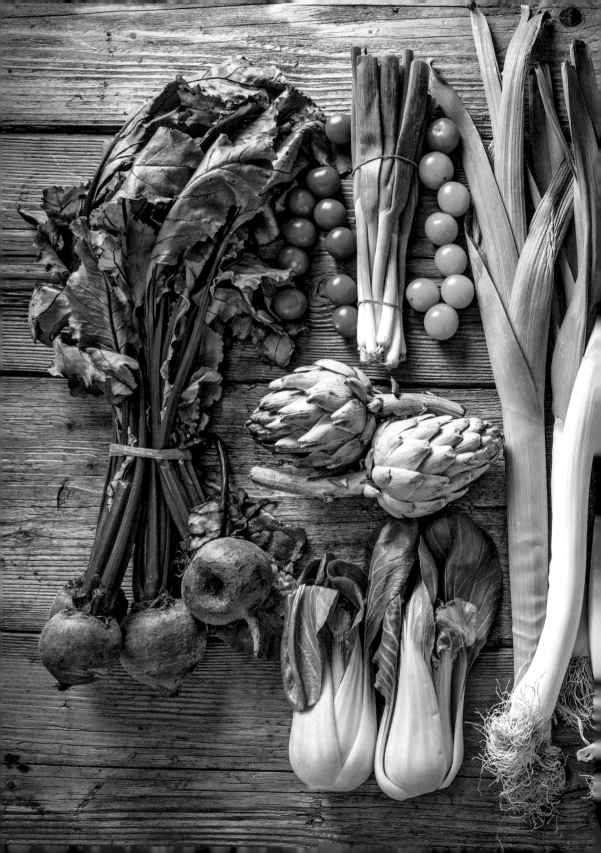

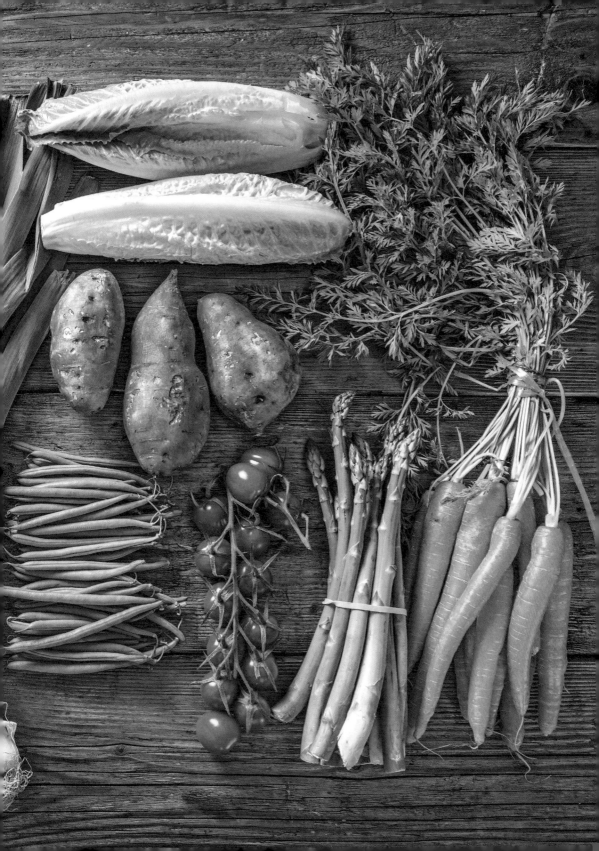

What Does the Color of Your Produce Indicate?

Phytochemicals are plant chemicals responsible for the color, flavor, and aroma of a fruit or vegetable, which is why color can be a good indicator of what's inside. Phytochemicals also provide health-supportive or disease-preventive properties, plus antioxidant and anti-inflammatory benefits. Scientists have discovered thousands of phytochemicals, and it's likely there are thousands more yet to be identified.

    Color does not tell all, though. A single piece of produce can contain thousands of different phytochemicals, and they ultimately work together to deliver their health benefits. So although the research around specific phytochemicals is interesting, they're always best consumed in whole foods rather than as supplements. The table below summarizes some of the more common and better-studied phytochemicals and the foods in which you're likely to find them.

Produce Color	Phytochemical	Possible Benefits	Sample Foods
Red	Lycopene	Supports cardiac and circulatory health; offers skin some protection from UV rays	Tomatoes, watermelon
Red	Anthocyanins	Protection against heart disease; anticarcinogenic	Cherries, cranberries, grapes, pomegranate
Red, orange, yellow	Alpha-carotene, beta-carotene	Supports healthy skin, eyesight, and cardiac health; converted to vitamin A in the body; antioxidant	Bell peppers, butternut squash, carrots, sweet potatoes
Red, orange, yellow	Lutein, zeaxanthin	Supports eye health	Bell peppers, mango, nectarines, papaya
Green	Chlorophyll, isothiocyanates, lutein, zeaxanthin	Supports liver and kidneys; supports detoxification; protects against cancer; supports eye health	Broccoli, collard greens, kale, spinach, turnip greens
Blue, purple, black	Anthocyanins	Protection against heart disease; anticarcinogenic	Blackberries, blueberries, eggplant, purple cabbage
White	Sulfur	Supports healthy skin, hair, nails, and muscles	Bok choy, Brussels sprouts, cauliflower, garlic, leeks, onions
Every color	Flavonoids	Antioxidant, lowers inflammation	Apples, bell peppers, broccoli, celery, onions, parsley, strawberries, tomatoes, watermelon

SUPPORTS REGULARITY & HEALTHY DIGESTION

Beyond just making you feel satisfied, the fiber in fresh produce supports healthy digestion and regularity.

Shared Concerns About Produce

There are common concerns when choosing produce. Here is what you should know.

PESTICIDES: THE ORGANIC VERSUS CONVENTIONAL DEBATE

Organic farming practices are becoming more common. Organic produce is more available than ever—and with good reason. Organic fruits and vegetables are better for you and the environment. Here's why.

First, they tend to be more nutritious. A review of 343 studies published in *The British Journal of Nutrition* found that organic foods contain higher concentrations of antioxidants and less of the toxic heavy metal cadmium than their conventional counterparts.

Second, supporting organic farms also means you're supporting a cleaner environment. Organic farming methods, such as crop rotation and natural fertilizers, are more sustainable in the long term. Chemicals used on conventional farms make their way into the air, soil, and water supply, spreading their contamination much farther than just your plate. They pose a serious threat to our ecosystems—and to the farm workers who spray them onto crops.

Finally, perhaps the most compelling reason to choose organic is to limit your personal exposure to agricultural chemicals, including pesticides and herbicides, many of which are toxic to the human body. For example, the average conventional apple is sprayed with more than forty-five different chemicals, including six known or suspected carcinogens, sixteen suspected hormone disruptors, five neurotoxins, and six developmental or reproductive toxins. (Learn more about which chemicals are on your produce at www.whatsonmyfood.org.)

Choosing organic means you're minimizing or limiting your exposure to these toxic chemicals. Although organic produce is a lot less contaminated than its conventional counterparts, "organic" doesn't necessarily mean the produce contains zero pesticide or herbicide residue. Pests, weeds, and diseases on organic farms are controlled primarily through natural, physical, mechanical, and biological metods, but when these practices aren't sufficient, a natural or synthetic substance may be used. Also, spraying from neighboring conventional farms is easily carried by the wind. Even if this were to happen, though, the produce would contain only a small amount of the chemicals—far less than if it were sprayed directly. And there is yet another reason to continue to choose organic: The more organic farms there are, the less likely it is that conventional blow over occurs.

In an ideal world, everything you eat would be organic—but in the real world, organic foods aren't always available or economical. That's why the Environmental Working Group's (EWG) annual Dirty Dozen Plus and Clean Fifteen lists are great

🕐 **Time-Saving Tip**

At the grocery store, an easy way to tell whether a food is organic is to look at the four- or five-digit code on its sticker. The numbers indicate how it was grown, as follows:

- Starts with a 4: conventionally grown
- Starts with a 9: organically grown

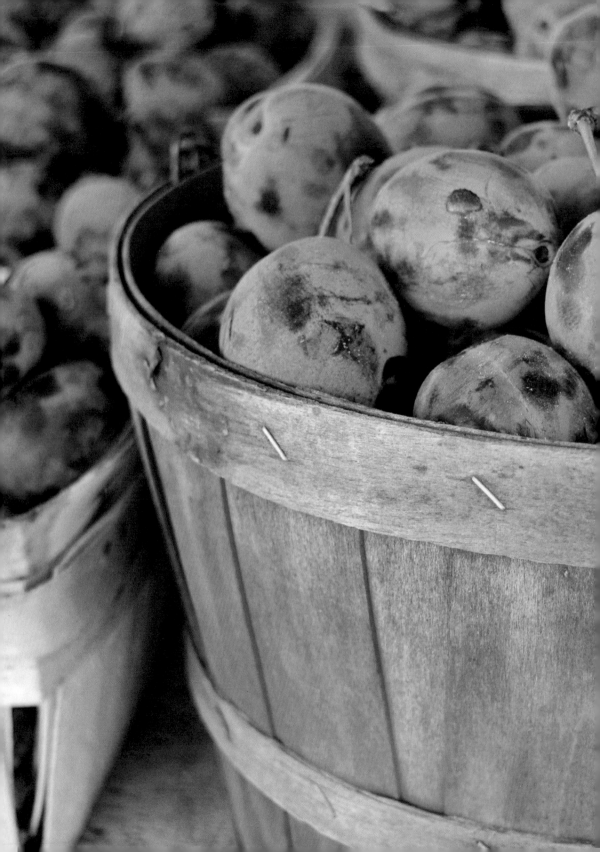

resources. They can help you decide which types of organic produce to invest in. Each year, the EWG tests thousands of produce samples to determine which fruits and vegetables contain the most—and most toxic—pesticides. The worst offenders land on the Dirty Dozen Plus list (from which you should consider buying organic), while the least-sprayed varieties make the Clean Fifteen list (from which you can feel good about buying conventional).

EWG's Clean Fifteen

The "Clean Fifteen" are the fruits and veggies sprayed with the smallest amount of agricultural chemicals—or with the least harmful ones. If you want to save money on your grocery bill, purchase the produce on this list in its conventional form. In general, the Clean Fifteen foods are those with a skin or peel that you remove before eating.

EWG's Dirty Dozen Plus

The "Dirty Dozen," on the other hand, is a list of foods that usually have the most pesticides sprayed on them and should therefore only be purchased as organic. In general, anything with a thin skin that you eat or without a protective outer layer should be purchased organic. In recent years, the EWG added the "plus" section to the list to include two foods that don't have the most pesticides overall but are treated with the most toxic and harmful ones: These foods should always be consumed in their organic forms, too, if you want to limit chemical exposure.

EATING SEASONALLY

In today's global economy, you can get practically any food at any time of the year. (For instance, you can get a pineapple in New York in the middle of winter.) So it's easy to forget that most food has a specific growing season.

Organic or Conventional Produce? How to Choose

ALWAYS BUY ORGANIC
EWG's Dirty Dozen Plus (2016)

- Strawberries
- Apples
- Nectarines
- Peaches
- Celery
- Grapes
- Cherries
- Spinach
- Tomatoes
- Sweet bell peppers
- Cherry tomatoes
- Cucumbers

Dirty Dozen Plus

- Hot peppers
- Kale/collard greens

OKAY TO BUY CONVENTIONAL
EWG's Clean Fifteen (2016)

- Avocado
- Sweet corn
- Pineapple
- Cabbage
- Sweet peas, frozen
- Onion
- Asparagus
- Mango
- Papaya
- Kiwi
- Eggplant
- Honeydew melon
- Grapefruit
- Cantaloupe
- Cauliflower

What's in Season?

Though local produce will vary according to region, the following information shows which foods are generally available each season in North America.

Spring	Summer	Fall	Winter	Always in Season
Apricot	Apricot	Apple	Grapefruit	Garlic
Broccoli	Avocado	Beet	Lemon	Onions
Cabbage	Bell peppers	Broccoli	Orange	Mushrooms
Green beans	Blackberries	Brussels	Pear	
Honeydew	Cantaloupe	sprouts	Potato	
melon	Cherries	Carrot	Sweet potato	
Lettuce	Corn	Cauliflower	Turnip	
Mango	Cucumber	Cranberries	Winter squash	
Peas	Eggplant	Figs		
Pineapple	Figs	Grapes		
Rhubarb	Grapefruit	Parsnip		
Spinach	Grapes	Pear		
Strawberries	Green beans	Persimmon		
	Honeydew	Pumpkin		
	melon	Sweet potato		
	Lima beans	Winter squash		
	Peach			
	Plum			
	Radish			
	Raspberries			
	Strawberries			
	Summer			
	squash			
	Tomato			
	Watermelon			
	Zucchini			

Food is information for our body, and it influences how our bodies react to the climate. It makes sense that heavy, hearty vegetables that warm us, such as beets and sweet potatoes, come into season during the cold fall and winter months, while, cooling, refreshing, cleansing juicy fruits or light vegetables—melons, berries, and zucchini—come into season in the hot summer months when we need cooling. In Eastern medicine, eating seasonally is believed to be important for optimal digestion and overall health.

WE'RE NOT EATING ENOUGH

We know eating fruits and vegetables adds nutrients to the diet; reduces the risk for heart disease, stroke, and some cancers; and helps manage body weight when consumed in place of more calorie-dense foods. But we're not eating nearly enough of them.

The U.S. *Dietary Guidelines for Americans* suggest that adults should consume at least one and a half to two cups of fruit (about 225 to 300 g depending on the fruit) and at least two to three cups of vegetables daily (weight varies depending on the vegetable). But only about one in ten Americans eats this amount. According to the National Cancer Institute, between 2007 and 2010, half of the U.S. population consumed less than one cup of fruit (about 150 g) and less than one and a half cups of vegetables (weight varies) daily; 76 percent did not meet the fruit intake recommendations; and 87 percent did not meet the vegetable intake recommendations.

Some researchers, functional medicine doctors, and even governments, however, believe the minimum fruit and vegetable intake should be higher for optimal health. A study published in the *Journal of Epidemiology and Community Health* suggests that people who eat "seven or more portions of fruit and vegetables daily have

> ### ❗ Expert Tip
>
> You can discover what produce is in season in your area each month by visiting www.sustainabletable.org or simply heading to your local farmers' market.

the lowest risk of mortality from any cause." The study assessed the habits of more than sixty-five thousand people aged thirty-five and older, through the 2001 to 2008 Health Surveys for England, plus several years of follow-up. Consuming at least seven servings was linked to a 42 percent lower risk of death from all causes; 31 percent lower risk of death from heart disease or stroke; and 25 percent lower risk of death from cancer, after excluding deaths within the first year of monitoring.

Kaiser Permanente, a leading health insurance company that also operates medical centers and hospitals, suggests that people eat an unlimited amount of vegetables—aiming for at least six servings of vegetables and two to four servings of fruit daily. Additionally, in Australia, the government promotes a "Go for 2+5" campaign, which suggests eating two servings of fruit and five servings of vegetables each day. So, use the information in the rest of this chapter to inspire you to increase your fruit and veggie intake!

BACTERIA

No matter how you plan to prepare your produce, always wash it first—even if it looks clean. There are many possible sources of (invisible) bacterial contamination, including contact with contaminated soil, irrigation water, manure, wildlife, or farm workers. Once contaminated, produce can harbor harmful bacteria, such as salmonella, *Listeria*, and E.coli, which can lead to foodborne illness. It can occur within twenty minutes and up to three days after ingesting tainted foods and lead to a variety of symptoms, including vomiting, diarrhea, abdominal pain, fever, headache, or body aches. And even if you plan to peel produce or eat only its inside—as with cantaloupe or avocado, for instance—you should still wash it: The knife you use to cut the food may transfer bacteria from the rind to the inside.

You don't need fancy vegetable washes, though. Washing produce with distilled water has been shown to remove as much as 98 percent of bacteria, which is comparable to or better than most commercial vegetable washes. Soaking or running under regular tap water should also do the trick.

Vegetables & Their Benefits

Loaded with vitamins, minerals, antioxidants, fiber, and even some protein, vegetables are like nature's medicine cabinet—and they may even be our lost fountain of youth! Veggies may not be on your list of favorite foods, but with the right recipes, they just may end up there. After reading about their benefits, I hope you'll be inspired to make a renewed effort to get them onto your plate.

And if you're scratching your head wondering what exactly you're going to eat on a diet of mostly produce, rest assured the possibilities are endless. While veggies may not look particularly appetizing on their own, with a little creativity (and the right recipes!), you can turn a head of cauliflower into a pizza crust or a sweet potato into a creamy, cheeseless mac and "cheese" sauce. And even without getting fancy, many vegetables become crave-worthy after simply roasting them with a little garlic powder and olive oil.

One of my secrets for getting kids and picky eaters to chow down on the good stuff is to use a spiralizer, an inexpensive kitchen gadget that turns vegetables, such as zucchini, sweet potatoes, and beets, into "noodles." For easy recipes that make veggies the stars of the show, head to www.mariamarlowe.com.

ANTI-AGING

Vegetables not only keep wrinkles at bay, but also keep your brain sharp and your memory intact. At least one study has shown that higher vegetable intake is associated with less skin wrinkling after sun exposure, while another has shown that diets rich in vitamin C, which is found in abundance in many vegetables including broccoli, bell peppers, and dark leafy greens, is associated with better skin aging and less wrinkling. In terms of brain health, nitrates in beets have been found to help increase blood flow to the brain, thereby improving mental performance, while higher vegetable intake in general—and of dark leafy greens in particular—has been associated with a slower rate of cognitive decline.

WEIGHT LOSS

Because of their high fiber, water, and nutrient content, the more veggies you eat, the less of everything else (such as snacks, desserts, and meat) you'll eat because they do such a good job of making you feel satisfied. Because they're naturally less calorie dense than most other foods, when you eat more of them and less of the other stuff, you're likely to see the numbers on the scale head south.

PROTECTION AGAINST CANCER

Study after study demonstrates the potential anticancer benefits of vegetables, particularly cruciferous vegetables, such as Brussels sprouts, cauliflower, kale, and broccoli. Numerous population studies have shown that a higher intake of cruciferous vegetables is associated with a lower risk of lung, stomach,

Cruciferous Vegetables

- Bok choy
- Broccoli
- Broccoli rabe
- Brussels sprouts
- Cabbage, green and red
- Cauliflower
- Collard greens
- Horseradish
- Kale
- Kohlrabi
- Mustard greens (and mustard seeds)
- Radish
- Rutabaga
- Tatsoi (Asian salad green)
- Turnip
- Watercress

colon, and rectal cancers. Their anticancer effect is believed to be due, at least in part, to their high glucosinolate content.

All cruciferous vegetables contain glucosinolates and the enzyme myrosinase, which, when combined through chopping or chewing, produces isothiocyanates (ITC). ITC are believed to be powerful cancer-fighting compounds: They've been shown to detoxify and remove carcinogens, kill cancer cells, and prevent tumors from growing.

To maintain their valuable health-promoting properties, avoid boiling or microwaving these vegetables, which may decrease ITC bioavailabilty (the amount of a substance that's absorbed by, and has an active effect on, the body). Eat them raw, steamed, or sautéed instead.

Vegetables & Their Concerns

Vegetables may be the most nutrient-dense food group, but they are not without their concerns, namely, gas and their effect on thyroid function. Here is what you should know:

GAS & BLOATING

You may find you have a little extra gas when you start incorporating more vegetables into your diet, but don't let that stand in your way! If you're not used to eating fiber-rich foods, it may take your body (and gut flora) time to adjust. Don't worry—they will. Raw veggies are notorious for causing excess gas, so if you're just starting to incorporate more into your diet, try adding cooked ones first and increase your fiber load gradually. In time, fiber-rich foods will actually improve your digestion. Drink plenty of water—at least eight glasses a day—to help the fiber do its job.

CRUCIFEROUS VEGETABLES & THYROID FUNCTION

Cruciferous vegetables have had a bit of an identity crisis in the past few years. They were mistakenly pegged as a real threat to thyroid health, particularly after an opinion piece in the *New York Times* made raw kale juice a scapegoat for the author's hypothyroidism. What the piece failed to mention, though, was that it is highly unlikely that kale—or other cruciferous vegetables, for that matter—could actually cause a thyroid issue, except in the case of iodine deficiency.

This confusion probably stems from a study carried out in the 1980s that suggested very high intakes of raw cruciferous vegetables caused hypothyroidism in animals. Further findings suggested that the breakdown products of glucosinolates, which are found in cruciferous vegetables, could interfere with thyroid hormone synthesis or compete with iodine for uptake by the thyroid.

Suggested Serving Size Guidelines for Vegetables	
Serving size	1 cup (weight varies) raw or cooked
Servings per day	Five or more
Frequency per week	Every day!

However, no human study has demonstrated that eating large amounts of cruciferous vegetables alone leads to issues with thyroid function.

The fact is that cruciferous vegetables are loaded with health-promoting properties, so there's no need for healthy individuals to stop consuming them.

Although iodine deficiency is rare, it does tend to be more common in plant-based eaters because iodine isn't found in many of these foods. Seaweed (kelp, dulse, wakame, or kombu) is the best source, followed by seafood and eggs. So keep eating your cruciferous veggies, but make sure you get enough iodine, too!

NIGHTSHADES

Nightshades are a class of plant-based foods that may spur inflammation and joint or digestive issues in people who are sensitive to them, particularly those with an auto-immune disease, a leaky gut, or arthritis. However, there isn't yet much scientific evidence to back this up or to make a strong case for avoiding these foods, which include potatoes (not sweet potatoes, though), tomatoes, eggplant, all types of hot and sweet peppers, (including spices such as cayenne pepper and paprika), and tomatillos. Despite this

lack of research, if you suffer from any of the conditions mentioned or another inflammatory condition, it can't hurt to remove these foods from your diet to determine whether it makes a difference for you.

Fruit & Its Benefits

Fruit is nature's candy. Juicy and sweet, it not only tastes good, it also does the body good. Like veggies, fruit is loaded with a variety of important vitamins, minerals, and antioxidants as well as fiber, water, and even healthy fats. Fruit makes a smart and healthy breakfast, snack, or dessert choice.

Most people tend to favor fruit over not-so-sweet veggies—but not everyone. If you're not terribly keen on fruit, know that experimentation is key: If you try different textures and preparations, you may discover a new favorite food. For example, you can turn frozen bananas into soft-serve ice cream with a high-speed blender or dates into chocolate truffles. You can also try fruit smoothies—or dip fresh fruit in melted, high-quality, naturally sweetened dark chocolate for a treat. These fruit-based desserts are also an excellent way to wean your palate off refined sugar without feeling deprived of your sweet fix.

ANTI-AGING

Fruit is high in a range of vitamins, minerals, and antioxidants, particularly vitamin C, which promotes collagen production and is necessary for youthful, wrinkle-resistant skin. Vitamin C is abundant in the skin, but as we age, vitamin C levels decrease and wrinkles appear. Two observational studies found that higher dietary intakes of vitamin C were associated with notable decreases in skin wrinkling and better skin appearance in general.

WEIGHT LOSS

Some people are afraid that fruit causes weight gain because it contains natural sugar. Numerous studies suggest the opposite, indicating fruit actually supports weight loss. In a review of more than twelve thousand food diaries, researchers at the USDA found that individuals of normal weight, including men, women, and children, consumed significantly more fruit than their overweight and obese counterparts. Another study published in the journal *Nutrition* found that when obese and overweight people simply added fruit to their diet, they lost significantly more weight than those who didn't.

Fruit & Its Concerns

Fruit may be delicious and healthy, but with the current backlash against sugar, it some-times is demonized for containing it. Here is what you need to know:

SUGAR

Yes, fruit contains sugar, but don't be scared of it. The fiber in fruit slows the absorption of sugar into the bloodstream, which means you won't get as high a blood sugar spike as you would if you ate an equal amount of sugar in a food lacking fiber, such as a candy bar. Plus, fruit is loaded with antioxidants and nutrients that support health, so cutting it out means cutting out these valuable benefits.

If you're concerned about a blood sugar spike in relatively high glycemic fruit, such as bananas or dates, pair the fruit with a high-protein food, such as raw nuts, to mini-mize the rise in blood sugar or simply choose lower sugar fruit, such as berries, instead.

FRUIT JUICE & DRIED FRUIT

While sugar in whole fruit doesn't present much cause for concern, fruit juice and dried

❗ Expert Tip

Suggested Serving Size Guidelines for Fruit	
Serving size	One medium-size piece of fruit; ½ cup (75 g) berries; 1 cup (160 g) melon
Servings per day	Two to four
Frequency per week	Every day!

fruit are a little different. Here's why. Freshly squeezed fruit juice does contain nutrients, but it also packs a lot more natural sugar than you'd normally consume if you ate the fruit whole and fresh. For instance, while you'd probably only eat one apple at a time, a glass of apple juice might contain 1 to 2 pounds (0.5 to 1 kg) of apples—without much, if any, of the fiber naturally found in the whole fruit.

Because fiber keeps blood sugar in check, avoid or limit the amount of fruit juice you drink, even the freshly squeezed kind. If you like to drink your fruit, a smoothie is a better option as it still contains fiber.

Similarly, dried fruit is high in sugar: As the water has been removed, it's easy to overeat. You may end up consuming the equivalent of three dried apples in place of a single fresh one—and, therefore, triple the amount of sugar you'd normally eat.

Produce: An In-Depth Look

The remainder of this chapter provides an in-depth look at the benefits of more than fifty types of produce and shows you how to select, store, and prepare them.

APPLE

As the old saying goes, an apple a day keeps the doctor away. Loaded with antioxidants, apples support cardiovascular and respiratory health and help keep blood sugar balanced. They've also been linked to a reduction in the risk of asthma and lung cancer.

Unfortunately, apples routinely end up at the top of the EWG's Dirty Dozen list (page 46)—a typical conventional apple contains up to forty-five different pesticides!

Selection: Always choose organic. Select apples with firm, unblemished skin. They shouldn't have bruises, feel spongy, or give at all when you press them gently.

Most nutritious varieties: mildly sweet varieties, including Braeburn, Cortland, Discovery, Gala, Granny Smith, Honeycrisp, Idared, McIntosh, Melrose, Ozark Gold, and Red Delicious

Least nutritious varieties: Pink Lady, Golden Delicious, Empire, Ginger Gold, and Elstar

Storage: Apples last up to ten times longer when stored in the refrigerator instead of on the countertop. Put them in your crisper drawer and set the humidity to high.

Preparation: Eat apples on their own (keep some in a bowl at the office); top with almond butter; or chop into oatmeal. You can also add them to smoothies or bake them and sprinkle with cinnamon for dessert. Because an unpeeled apple contains more fiber, vitamins, and phytonutrients than a peeled one, choose organic and eat the skin.

Flesh should feel firm, not soft or spongy.

Avoid fruit with blemishes.

ARTICHOKE

At first glance, artichokes may not seem like a nutritional powerhouse—but they are! They're surprisingly high in antioxidants and fiber (a whopping ten grams, or 41 percent, of the recommended daily value [DV] of fiber per artichoke), which are largely responsible for their cardiac benefits. They're also high in inulin, a prebiotic that supports a healthy gut, and folate, a critical nutrient that prevents birth defects, blood disease, and possibly even cancer. One artichoke provides 27 percent of the DV of folate.

Selection: Choose larger artichokes that have densely packed leaves: They'll have larger hearts than the slim, pointed chokes. Artichokes with a thorn at the end of each leaf will have a nuttier flavor. Varieties without the thorns have softer flesh.

Artichokes do require about an hour of cooking time, so a faster but equally nutritious option is packaged artichoke hearts. They are still high in antioxidants and low in calories. Ideally, artichoke hearts should be purchased in glass jars instead of cans, which can leach chemicals. Choose artichokes packed in water, olive oil, or a spice mixture.

If you see purple artichokes, grab them. They contain the cancer-fighting compounds *anthocyanins*, making them even more nutritious.

Storage: Keep refrigerated in the crisper drawer and eat within three days: Artichokes spoil quickly. Artichoke hearts, on the other hand, have a longer shelf life.

Preparation: Steam artichokes to retain the most antioxidants or simmer in water. Use artichoke hearts as a snack or a topping on salad.

Leaves should be densely packed, not open.

Choose artichokes that are large in size.

The tips should be tightly closed.

Stems should be straight, not bent.

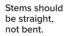 **Money-Saving Tip**

How to Keep Producer Fresher, Longer

Make and use a micro-perforated bag, which lets small amounts of air in and out of the bag. Some produce will last days longer in a micro-perforated bag. To make one, use a pin to prick evenly spaced holes in a resealable plastic bag (ten holes for a quart [946 ml] bag, twenty holes for anything larger). You can use (and reuse!) this bag to extend the shelf life of a variety of produce, particularly lettuce and dark leafy greens such as kale and broccoli.

ASPARAGUS

Asparagus is an excellent source of vitamin K and folate (offering 22 percent and 27 percent DV, respectively, per cup, or 134 g) as well as inulin, which supports digestive health. What's most intriguing, though, is that it's the best food source of *glutathione*, a detoxifying antioxidant that breaks down carcinogens and may aid in preventing and reversing certain types of cancer.

Selection: Fresh asparagus not only tastes better, it also retains more of its nutritional value. Its nutrients do deteriorate quickly, though, so only buy what you'll consume within a day or two. Look for thin, tender spears that are dark green, shiny, and straight, not bent. The tips should be tightly closed and green or purplish in color. The cut end of the stalk should be smooth and moist.

Skip white asparagus, which is simply green asparagus that's been buried in soil so it never sees the light of day. It's tougher and has only one-seventh the antioxidants it has when grown normally.

You'll find the best asparagus at farmers' markets. Seek out farmers who display theirs on ice: These will be the most tender because delayed chilling toughens them.

Storage: Asparagus is best eaten on the day of purchase, as it loses nutrients and flavor rapidly. If you plan to keep it for more than a day, refrigerate it in a micro-perforated bag (see at left) in the crisper drawer. It will last only a few days, at most.

Preparation: The best preparation for asparagus is steaming: It takes five minutes and increases its antioxidant value by 30 percent.

AVOCADO

Avocado is loaded with fiber—one medium avocado provides 40 percent of your DV. One avocado also provides a hefty dose of key nutrients, including 39 percent of your DV of vitamin K, which supports bone health and proper blood clotting, and 20 percent of your DV for vitamins E and C, which support beautiful skin. What's more, healthy fats from avocados help you absorb the fat-soluble vitamins in other foods, making them an excellent topping for leafy green salads. There's no need to fear avocado: Eat up!

Selection: Choose Haas avocados—the ones that turn blackish when ripe and have a rough, alligator-like skin. Haas is the most nutrient-dense and best-tasting variety. Sometimes you'll also see green avocados with smooth, shiny skin, which can be any of a number of different varieties. To choose one, look for those with deep dark green, almost blackish, skin. These will be ripe. Avoid any with soft spots, air pockets, or a pit that seems to be rolling around inside. Next, remove the little center stem nub on the top. If green flesh is revealed, it's fresh. If it's brown or moldy, the avocado is bad and will be brown inside.

Most nutritious varieties: Haas avocados, green avocados

Least nutritious varieties: Florida avocados

Storage: Avocados should be stored on the countertop and consumed within a day or two when ripe. You can throw a ripe avocado into the fridge to slowly decay, but it will only last an additional day or two, at best. Cut avocados brown quickly: To slow browning, always store the half with the pit. The most effective way to prevent browning is to store the cut half in a small glass container with coarsely chopped onion in the bottom (so the skin of the avocado, not the flesh, touches the onion), seal it with a tight-fitting lid, and then refrigerate it. The onion's volatile oils are powerful antioxidants that prevent browning.

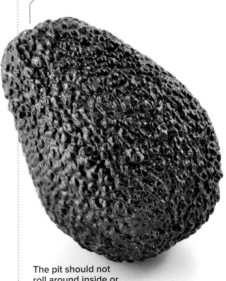

Remove stem nub at the top; if it is green underneath, it is fresh.

The pit should not roll around inside or feel loose.

For guacamole, submerge the pits inside the mixture to slow oxidation. To store it, put a piece of plastic wrap over the bowl and press it down on top of the guacamole—removing any air to prevent the top from browning—and then refrigerate.

Preparation: The greatest concentration of nutrients is in the slightly darker green flesh just below the skin, so be sure it ends up on your plate and not in the garbage. The simplest way is to score it and scoop it out with a spoon. (Alternatively, you can peel the skin first.) Here's how:

- Cut the avocado lengthwise around the pit, producing two long avocado halves still connected in the middle by the seed.

- Take hold of both halves and twist them in opposite directions until they naturally separate. At this point, use a knife to remove the seed. (Carefully whack it with a chef's knife so the blade gets lodged in the pit; twist and pull lightly to remove; and then bang the handle of the knife on the edge of the sink to get the pit off the knife.)

- Use the knife to cut each half lengthwise to produce long quartered sections of avocado.

- Use your thumb and index finger to grip the edge of the skin on each quarter and peel it off, just as you'd do with a banana skin. The final result is a peeled avocado that contains most of that dark green outer flesh that's so rich in antioxidants.

Spread smashed avocado on toast; chop it and add it to salads; or make it into guacamole. You could also slice one open, sprinkle with a little salt and some red pepper flakes, and eat it with a spoon for a satisfying snack.

Water-Soluble versus Fat-Soluble Vitamins

In general, there are two types of vitamins: water soluble and fat soluble.

Water-soluble vitamins dissolve in water, which is why you should avoid boiling vegetables: The water-soluble vitamins will end up in the water you discard. Once ingested, these vitamins are absorbed and excreted readily: They aren't stored in the body.

Water-soluble vitamins include all B vitamins—folate, thiamine, riboflavin, niacin , pantothenic acid, biotin, B_6, and vitamin B_{12}—and vitamin C.

Fat-soluble vitamins dissolve in fat and need to be consumed with fat to be absorbed. Therefore, foods containing fat-soluble vitamins, such as salad greens, should always be eaten with some sort of healthy fat, such as olive oil, avocado, nuts, or seeds.

Fat-soluble vitamins include vitamins A, D, E, and K.

BANANA

Bananas are an excellent source of vitamin B_6 (22 percent DV per banana) and a good source of fiber and minerals—especially potassium. Potassium, which is found in many vegetables and fruits, plays a key role in a variety of bodily processes and supports heart, bone, and muscle health.

Selection: Sometimes, green bananas don't ripen correctly at home—or take up to a week to do so—so choose yellow bananas with zero to minimal green at the top and be sure they're free of brown spots, soft spots, and bruises. Ideally, choose organic, as they tend to taste better.

Storage: Store bananas on the countertop. They will develop brown spots and get sweeter as they ripen. You can refrigerate ripe bananas to slow spoiling, but if you're not going to eat them within a day or two, freeze them for use in desserts and smoothies instead. Simply peel, split in half, and place them in a zip-top bag, and put into the freezer. Don't refrigerate unripened bananas: They won't ripen properly. Their skin will turn black, and they won't become sweet.

Preparation: Eat them on their own; add them to smoothies; slice and sprinkle with cinnamon and almond butter; or dip them in dark chocolate. You can also use frozen bananas to make nondairy ice cream. The riper the banana, the higher its glycemic load. So, sprinkle a ripe banana with cinnamon or spread it with almond butter if you're concerned about keeping your blood sugar in check.

Bananas should be yellow, not green.

Avoid brown spots or bruises.

❗ Expert Tip

If you go overboard on salty junk food and find yourself bloated, consider eating potassium-rich foods to reduce water retention. In addition to bananas, avocados, beans, dark leafy greens, and sweet potatoes are good sources.

Greens should be bright green and crisp, not limp.

Select beets with greens still attached.

BEETS & BEET GREENS

Brightly colored red and yellow beets are loaded with antioxidants. Interestingly, though, beet greens, which many people throw away, have a delicious, sweet, spinach-like flavor and more antioxidants than the roots themselves. They're on a nutritional par with kale.

Athletes may want to add more beets to their diet: Research shows that beets and beet juice can improve performance by increasing blood flow to muscles and reducing the amount of oxygen required during exercise. This means that drinking or eating beets before working out allows you to exercise harder and longer. Likewise, beets increase blood flow to the brain, which may slow the progression of dementia and keep the brain in tip-top shape.

Selection: Choose beets with their greens still attached when you can find them: They'll be fresher. The greens should be brightly colored and firm, not limp.

Storage: If you buy beets with their greens, store them separately. Chop off the stems about one inch (2.5 cm) above the root. Greens should be stored in a micro-perforated bag (see page 56) and will last only one to two days. Roots go unwrapped into the crisper drawer where they will last one to two weeks.

Preparation: Roast or steam beets for a warm side dish or salad topper. For a cold preparation, grate them over a salad.

For beet greens: Use the entire top, including the greens and stems. Slice into quarter-inch (6 mm) strips and sauté with garlic and olive oil.

Avoid strawberries with white tops.

BERRIES
STRAWBERRIES, BLUEBERRIES, BLACKBERRIES & RASPBERRIES

Antioxidant-rich berries are easy-to-find superfoods. They may even help reduce arterial plaque; soothe inflammation; and even reverse age-related mental decline. Blackberries and blueberries, in particular, contain phytonutrients that may aid in cancer prevention. Though all berries provide fiber, raspberries and blackberries are a particularly good source, providing more than 30 percent DV per cup (about 130 g).

Selection: Always choose organic as berries often end up high on the EWG's Dirty Dozen list (page 46). Select berries that look firm and plump. Avoid any that look shriveled, soft, moldy, or like they're leaking. Strawberries should be completely red—not red at the bottom and white at the top, which is a sign they're less ripe, less nutritious, and less tasty!

Storage: Berries are highly perishable and rarely last longer than a few days or, at most, a week. Eat within a few days of purchase or refrigerate in the crisper drawer.

To help them last a few days longer, immediately give them a vinegar bath to kill any mold spores or bacteria. Mix one part white vinegar with three parts water in a bowl and swirl the berries around in this mixture for five minutes. Then drain, rinse well, and dry the berries thoroughly with paper towels before placing them in a paper towel–lined ventilated container. (Rinse and use the plastic one the berries came in.) Finally, return them to the fridge. (This doesn't work well for raspberries, though: It tends to make them mushy.)

Preparation: Eat berries on their own or add to oatmeal, smoothies, or salads. Interestingly, cooked blueberries happen to be more nutritious than raw ones, as the heat increases antioxidant levels. So, use them to make jams, syrups, or healthier desserts.

Avoid berries that are soft or shriveled in texture.

⊗ Money-Saving Tip

Does your produce spoil before you get a chance to eat it? Try FreshPaper produce saver sheets—all natural, spice-infused sheets that keep fruit and veggies fresh two to four times longer than they'd last on their own. They're easy to use: Simply slip one into your fruit bowl, fridge bowl, berry carton, or salad bag. Moldy berries will be history! Find them online at fenugreen.com or other online retailers, such as Amazon.

BOK CHOY

Bok choy is a highly nutritious cruciferous vegetable abundant in vitamins A, C, and K (providing 144 percent, 74 percent, and 72 percent DV, respectively, per cup, shredded, or 70 g) and minerals, including calcium (16 percent DV), potassium (18 percent DV), and iron (10 percent DV). It has anti-inflammatory properties and is being studied for its possible role in cancer prevention. At just twenty calories per cup (70 g), bok choy is a food you should consider adding to your diet.

Avoid browning or yellowing leaves.

Selection: Look for bok choy with firm, bright green leaves and moist, hardy stems. The leaves should look fresh, not wilted, and be free from signs of browning or yellowing.

Storage: Whether you choose regular-size bok choy, which is great for salads, or baby bok choy, which is more tender and perfect for stir-frying, store it in your refrigerator's crisper drawer in a sealed plastic bag with as much air removed as possible. It will keep for about four to five days.

Preparation: Chop bok choy into bite-size pieces to use in salads or steam, braise, roast, or sauté it as part of a veggie medley. It's most commonly found in Asian stir-fry recipes.

Stems should be moist, hardy, and vivid in color.

BROCCOLI

Cruciferous veggies, such as broccoli, contain glucosinolates, compounds being studied for their anticancer potential. One small but compelling human study has linked sulforaphane, a molecule found readily in broccoli and other cruciferous vegetables, to decreased autism spectrum symptoms. And a 2013 animal study linked that same molecule to reducing cognitive decline and slowing the progression of Parkinson's disease—although both studies are small and preliminary.

Still, it's high in fiber and a variety of nutrients, including vitamins C and K, making broccoli an easy and accessible superfood.

The buds of the floret should be tightly closed.

The stem should be firm and crisp, not rubbery.

Selection: Broccoli florets should be dark green and have tightly closed buds. Avoid any with large amounts of white, yellow, or light green. If it has only a little bit of a color change, that's okay. You can just chop it off at home. The stalk should be firm, not rubbery.

Storage: If you're not going to eat your broccoli within a day or two of purchase, store it in a micro-perforated bag (page 56) and it will last about a week. Remember that produce typically loses its nutrient value the longer you store it.

Preparation: Raw broccoli has up to twenty times the amount of sulforaphane (the compound largely connected to its anticancer properties) than cooked broccoli. Try dipping raw florets in tapenade or guacamole. For cooked preparations, roast it for ten to fifteen minutes in a 400°F (200°C, or gas mark 6) oven, steam it for about four minutes, or quickly sauté it with garlic and olive oil.

BRUSSELS SPROUTS

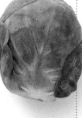

The leaves should be tightly packed, not loose.

Avoid sprouts that are yellow or feel rubbery.

If taste weren't reason enough to eat these small, cabbage-like sprouts, here's another: Research shows they may be a powerful protector against cancer. They're most closely associated with preventing cancers of the bladder, breast, colon, lung, prostate, and ovaries. Numerous studies have shown that compounds found in Brussels sprouts and other cruciferous vegetables have the ability to halt cancer cells in test tubes and they've even been found to induce cancer cell death in human studies. They aid in detoxification and provide an array of nutrients and antioxidants, including the B vitamins, iron, calcium, and more than 100 percent DV of vitamins C and K.

Selection: Look for bright green sprouts with tightly packed leaves. Avoid any that feel rubbery, have lots of loose leaves, or look yellow. At the farmers' market, you'll often find them still attached to the stalk—it doesn't get any fresher than that!

Storage: Always keep Brussels sprouts refrigerated and eat them soon after purchase—ideally within two or three days, as they lose their freshness quickly. However, if you store them in a plastic bag in your crisper drawer, they may last a week or more. If you purchased them on a stalk, wrap the bottom of the stem in a wet paper towel, put a plastic bag around it, and break the sprouts off as needed.

Preparation: Rinse and trim the stems just before use. Cut into quarters, dress with your favorite oil and spices, and roast in a 450°F (230°C, or gas mark 8) oven for thirty to thirty-five minutes, tossing occasionally. You could also steam them for no more than six to eight minutes (any longer and they'll lose taste and nutrients). To serve, toss with olive oil, salt, and pepper or a vinaigrette. Whatever you do, avoid boiling them: Aside from subpar texture and flavor, you'll lose much of their B vitamins and vitamin C.

❗ Expert Tip

Certain people are highly sensitive to bitter tastes, so they end up shunning some of the healthiest foods, such as Brussels sprouts or kale, because of it. The trick to making these foods palatable for these individuals is to mask their bitter flavor. You can do that by pairing them with whole-grain Dijon mustard. They'll go down much easier—even for picky eaters!

CABBAGE

Cabbage tends to be overshadowed by more popular veggies such as kale, but nutritionally, it's still a superstar. Research has shown that cabbage helps lower cholesterol, supports detoxification, and contains nutrients of potential benefit to our stomach and intestinal lining.

As a member of the cruciferous vegetable family, it contains the same cancer-inhibiting compounds and anti-inflammatory benefits already discussed. It's rich in fiber, antioxidants, vitamins K and C, and the B vitamins.

Selection: You'll find three types of cabbage at your grocery store: green; red (which looks more like a deep purple); and savoy. All cabbage is highly nutritious, but the purplish-red cabbage is especially good for you: It boasts a variety of additional antioxidants, including anthocyanins, which exhibit strong disease-fighting potential.

Choose cabbage heads that are firm and heavy. The outer leaves should be shiny, crisp, and free from major cracks and blemishes. Only a few of the outer leaves should be loose. The rest should be tightly packed. Avoid preshredded cabbage; it loses its vitamin C content quickly once cut.

Storage: Place cabbage in a plastic bag and into the crisper drawer of your refrigerator. Red and green cabbage should last about two weeks this way, and savoy will last about one week. Once cut, use it within a few days to retain the most vitamin C.

Preparation: Cut the bottom core off the cabbage and then slice it into quarters. From there, you can shred it on a mandoline, in a food processor, or by hand with a knife. Add it raw to salads, steam it, sauté it, braise it, or throw it in the pressure cooker. Only cook it until just soft—overcooking reduces many of its nutritional benefits. Research suggests steaming cabbage increases its potential to lower cholesterol.

Purple and red cabbage have the most antioxidants.

Outer leaves should be shiny and crisp, not dull and limp.

⏱ Time-Saving Tip

Pressure cook your veggies. A pressure cooker is in invaluable kitchen tool. It not only cooks vegetables incredibly quickly, it also intensifies their flavor and retains more nutrients than other cooking methods. For example, it takes about an hour to braise cabbage in the oven and only fifteen minutes in the pressure cooker. And it takes about fifteen minutes to roast broccoli; five minutes to steam it; and just two minutes to pressure cook it.

65

CANTALOUPE

Cantaloupe is a juicy summer melon that provides high amounts of vitamins A and C (108 percent and 98 percent of your DV, respectively, per cup of cubes [160 g]) as well as antioxidant and anti-inflammatory benefits. Plus, it's loaded with water, so it fills you up quickly and helps keep you hydrated. Between its vitamin and water content, cantaloupe is a true "beauty food" that supports clear, glowing skin.

Selection: When buying a whole cantaloupe, look for those that feel heavy for their size and have no dents, fissures, or mold. The stem end of the fruit should have a slight depression. If it has a stub, it was probably picked too soon and won't ripen and develop its flavor correctly. Sniff the fruit near the stem depression. It should smell sweet, like cantaloupe, indicating it's ripe. If it doesn't smell, it will need a day or two to ripen.

For precut melon, choose those with the deepest orange flesh. If it looks like the melon is resting in a lot of water, it probably isn't fresh.

Storage: Cantaloupe will continue to ripen on the countertop. A ripe melon will last up to five days in the crisper drawer of your refrigerator. Once cut, cover it with plastic wrap and refrigerate.

Preparation: Even though you won't be eating the rind, scrub cantaloupe well under running water before you cut it: Its netted skin can pick up and harbor bacteria from the soil or during harvesting, packing, storage, or transport, including salmonella and deadly E. coli. To eat it, cut it in half, scoop out the seeds and pulp, and fill with berries for an antioxidant-rich breakfast. Or, simply chop the flesh to enjoy it on its own or add it to smoothies or salads.

The stem end should have a slight depression, not a stub.

CARROT

The humble carrot is a nutritional superstar. Its bright orange color is an indicator of its high vitamin A content (113 percent DV per cup, or 130 g), which supports eye and skin health. A ten-year cohort study from the Netherlands found that participants who consumed the largest amount of deep orange produce had the lowest risk of cardiovascular disease (CVD), which is currently the number one killer globally. Carrot consumption, in particular, seemed to offer the greatest benefits: For every quarter-cup (33 g) increase in carrot intake, participants lowered their risk of CVD by 32 percent (increased consumption of other fruits and vegetables didn't seem to result in any significant reduction). Carrots are low in calories and high in fiber, making them a filling snack when served on their own or with a healthy dip.

Selection: Choose firm carrots that aren't rubbery, ideally with their green tops intact as this is a sign of freshness. You can even eat the tops raw in salads or cooked if you like, though they have a bitter taste. If you can't find them, don't worry: Those with the tops removed are still okay. If you see purple, red, or yellow carrots, grab them. They're heirloom varieties, loaded with extra antioxidants.

Storage: Cut off the green stems (and use right away) before refrigerating the carrots to preserve their moisture. Stored in a sealed plastic bag in the crisper drawer, they should last four to five weeks.

Preparation: Eat carrots raw dipped into hummus, guacamole, or tapenade; or roast with a little olive oil to bring out their sweetness and increase their nutrients and anticancer compounds.

Carrots with the greens attached are the freshest.

Carrots should be firm, not rubbery.

CAULIFLOWER

With all the dazzling greens, oranges, and reds in the produce aisle, it's easy to overlook that stark white head of cauliflower. Despite its bland color, cauliflower is highly nutritious. As another member of the cruciferous vegetable family, it aids in detoxification, reduces inflammation, and also contains a variety of compounds found to aid in cancer prevention. At a measly 28 calories per cup cooked (124 g)—but a whopping 12 percent DV of fiber and 92 percent DV of vitamin C!—you can feel good about chowing down on this vegetable.

Selection: Choose a head with no spots, speckles, bruises, or traces of mold. Don't buy any with a boxy or "shaved" appearance, which is a sign that the grocery store removed moldy patches. If you see bright purple, yellow, or green cauliflower, grab it. These varieties are loaded with extra antioxidants. Plus, they look so striking they add a wow factor to any plate.

Storage: Cauliflower will last about one week in the crisper drawer.

Preparation: Sauté or steam for no more than ten minutes to maintain nutritional integrity, crispness, and flavor. You can also roast cauliflower, either chopped in florets or as cauliflower "steaks:" That is, in one-inch-thick (2.5 cm) slabs, a cooking style that's become trendy in vegetable-centric restaurants. Roast at a high temperature, 400°F to 450°F (200°C, or gas mark 6, to 230°C, or gas mark 8) and coat with a little olive oil and your favorite spices. It's great in curry or tomato-sauce dishes as well. You can eat cauliflower raw as crudité with a healthy dip if you like, but it's generally easier to digest when cooked. As with all vegetables, avoid boiling, which generally turns your delicious produce into waterlogged, unpalatable mush.

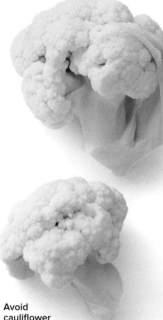

Don't buy cauliflower that has a "shaved" or boxy appearance.

Avoid cauliflower with spots, bruises, or mold.

CELERY

Crisp, crunchy celery isn't just a low-cal snack; it's also loaded with antioxidants and phytonutrients. Celery helps reduce inflammation, particularly in the digestive tract, and supports cardiovascular health. At a barely there six calories per stalk, grab a bowl of hummus or guacamole and get dipping!

Selection: Always choose organic as celery is ranked number 5 on the *EWG*'s Dirty Dozen list. Stalks should be firm, not rubbery or limp.

Storage: Store celery in your refrigerator's crisper drawer and for maximum nutrients, consume within five to seven days.

Preparation: Dip organic celery sticks in hummus, tapenade, guacamole, or almond butter as a snack. Chop and use as part of a base for soups and stews, along with carrots and onions.

Always buy organic.

Stalks should be crisp, not rubbery or limp.

CORN

Corn is an American staple, and no summer barbeque would be complete without it. But there's a catch: Modern corn varieties are notorious for being high in sugar, low in nutrients, and genetically modified.

There are, however, a number of old-fashioned, mildly sweet varieties and colorful heirloom varieties you can choose if you're looking for a healthier way to include corn in your diet.

Selection: Always choose organic to avoid genetically modified crops and agricultural chemicals. Pull back the husks or squeeze the ear to feel the kernels: They should be closely spaced, firm, and round. Look for tightly wrapped husks and moist stems.

Most nutritious varieties: Yellow corn is the most nutritious type of corn you'll easily find at your local grocer. It has more vitamin A and antioxidants than white corn. Black, blue, purple, and red varieties are even more nutritious, but they're typically only available at specialty grocers and farmers' markets.

Least nutritious varieties: White corn, pale yellow corn, or corn with a combination of white and pale yellow kernels are all super-sweet varieties that can contain as much as 40 percent sugar.

Storage: Refrigerate corn in its husks and cook within one to two days for the most nutrition and flavor.

Preparation: There are other more nutritious fruits and veggies on the market, so consume corn sparingly. Instead of boiling corn, which renders it less nutritious, steam it on the stovetop after removing the husks and silk. You can also grill corn with or without its husk. Dress it in lime juice and chili powder or hot sauce.

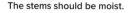

Kernels should be closely spaced and round in shape.

The stems should be moist.

CUCUMBER

The crisp, cool cucumber is mostly water, making it a filling low-calorie snack or salad topping. Cucumbers contain a variety of antioxidants and minerals and offer anti-inflammatory benefits, both when consumed and used on the skin. They may ease inflammation internally and may also help reduce skin puffiness, which is why they're sometimes placed over your eyes at spas. Most notably, they contain fisetin, an antioxidant that plays an important role in brain health, including improving memory and protecting brain cells from age-related decline.

Selection: Choose organic cucumbers with bright or dark green, firm skin. Avoid any with soft spots or wrinkled ends.

Storage: While usually sold refrigerated, cucumbers are best stored on the countertop at room temperature, according to research by scientists at the University of California, Davis. As it turns out, the refrigerator actually speeds their demise, turning them into watery, pitted logs after just three days. If you like your cukes cold, refrigerate them briefly before using or be sure to consume them within three days.

Preparation: Slice into spears for dipping in tapenade, hummus, or guacamole. Slice into rounds for salads; juice or blend them to make cucumber water; or add them to a smoothie for a hydrating drink.

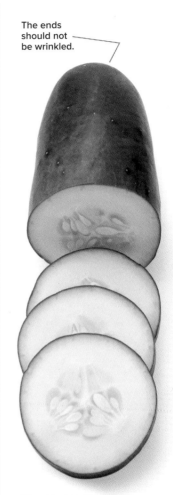

The ends should not be wrinkled.

The skin should be dark green and firm.

DATE

This mineral- and fiber-rich fruit also happens to be one of the sweetest, making dates an excellent alternative to packaged desserts and candy. Date-sweetened desserts and smoothies will satisfy any sweet tooth—no need for refined sugar.

Selection: When dates are in season, typically between September and March, you'll be able to find them fresh on the vine in the produce section. They'll be a little wrinkled, but they shouldn't be hard or dried out or have white crystals on them (which is an indicator that the sugar is moving to the surface and they're not as fresh). Choose plump dates with slightly glossy skin. When they're not in season, you can usually buy dried dates in the bulk section of your grocery store.

Storage: Store both fresh and dried dates in an airtight container in the refrigerator. Fresh dates should last at least a month, and dried dates can last up to a year when stored this way. If you keep dried dates in your pantry, they should last up to six months.

Preparation: Dates contain a large center pit, so pull them apart and remove the stem before biting into one. If they get too dry, you can rehydrate them by soaking in warm water for ten to fifteen minutes. You can eat dates on their own, but they're extremely sweet, and mixing them with other ingredients mellows them a bit. Stuff them with a savory filling, such as nuts; blend them into smoothies; or use them as a sweetener in healthy desserts, such as chocolate truffles or a nut-based raw pie-crust. To ease a blood sugar spike, get in the habit of pairing them with a protein-rich food, such as nuts.

The skin should be slightly glossy and free of white crystals.

Fruit should be soft, not hard or dry.

EGGPLANT

Eggplant is best known as the star of eggplant Parmesan and ratatouille, a classic French dish. Its deep, dark, purplish-black skin is an indicator of the presence of anthocyanins, potent anticancer phytonutrients. Other than that, though, it's not a particularly high source of vitamins or fiber, although research has connected eggplant consumption with brain and heart health. According to widespread anecdotal reports, people who suffer from inflammatory conditions, such as arthritis or fibroids, may find that consuming nightshade vegetables, including eggplant, may cause a flare in inflammatory symptoms—although little scientific evidence supports this claim. Still, if you notice a flare in your inflammatory symptoms after eating eggplant, consider eliminating it from your diet to see if you find relief.

Selection: Choose eggplants that are firm and heavy for their size. Skin should be smooth, shiny, and free of bruises.

Storage: Eggplants are delicate and perishable. Store whole in a plastic bag in the crisper drawer of your refrigerator. Be careful not to crush them under other vegetables. Eat within about four days if you purchased it at a supermarket or seven days if you got it at a farmers' market.

Preparation: Eggplant doesn't have a strong flavor on its own, so it can be used in a variety of preparations. Try your hand at making ratatouille, the classic French vegetable stew; slice it and use it instead of pasta in an inventive lasagna dish; or simply bake, roast, or steam it as you wish. It also goes well in curries and tomato-based sauces.

Skin should be smooth and free of bruises.

It should feel firm and heavy for its size.

FENNEL

Fennel is crunchy and slightly sweet, with a licorice or anise flavor. It's typically used in Mediterranean cuisines and is delicious raw or cooked. Fennel contains a variety of nutrients that support bone health, including calcium, magnesium, and vitamin K, and is a good source of both fiber and vitamin C.

Selection: Fennel should smell lightly of licorice. Look for bulbs that are clean, firm, and solid, with no signs of splitting or bruising. The bulb should be white or pale green, and the green stalks should stick straight up. Avoid fennel with signs of flowering, which indicates it's past its prime.

Storage: Store in the crisper drawer of your refrigerator, where it should last about four days.

Preparation: The entire fennel bulb—base, stalks, and leaves—is edible. Most recipes call for the bulb, but the stalks go well in soups or stews, and the leaves can be used just like fresh herbs. Try slicing the raw bulb into salads or cook it any way you please: sauté, roast, braise—or blend it into a soup.

Avoid fennel with signs of flowering.

Bulbs should be clean and firm with no sign of splitting or bruising.

FIG

Fresh figs are extremely delicate, so it's often hard to find them on the east coast of the United States (they're primarily grown in the west). Unlike most other fruits and veggies, fresh figs are still only available seasonally, from summer to early fall, although it's easier to find them dried. If you can find them fresh, snap them up as a gorgeous breakfast or salad topping or as a delicious snack on their own. There's nothing quite like biting into a fresh fig, which is actually an inverted flower. They're thought to be an aphrodisiac and according to legend, were one of Cleopatra's favorite foods. Healthwise, figs contain a variety of minerals, but are probably best known as a quick remedy for constipation, thanks to their high fiber content of about two grams, or 7 percent DV, per fig.

Selection: Figs have a short season—June through September—so when you see them fresh, buy them. They should be plump with smooth skin. Avoid any with bruising or soft spots. There are many varieties of figs, and they range in color from black to purple to green.

You can usually find dried figs in the bulk section year-round. Choose organic to avoid sulfites, a preservative that can cause an adverse reaction in some people.

Storage: Figs are highly perishable, so only buy what you'll eat in a day or two (which shouldn't be a problem, thanks to their unique taste and texture). Refrigerate ripe figs in a shallow, covered bowl, so they don't get crushed or pick up food odors. Underripe figs should be stored on the counter away from direct sunlight. Dried figs will last in a sealed container in a cool, dark place, such as the pantry, for months.

Preparation: Eat figs on their own for a tasty treat or slice them into oatmeal, parfaits, or salads. You can stuff them with walnuts or a savory filling; use them in desserts; make fig jam; or add them to smoothies.

Texture should be soft with firm skin.

Avoid figs with bruising or overly soft spots.

75

GARLIC

Garlic may leave you with stinky breath and fingers, but these are a small price to pay for its health benefits. When it's chopped or crushed, two chemicals in garlic, alliinase and alliin, combine to produce a compound called allicin, which exhibits antioxidant, antibacterial, antiviral, anticlotting, and anticancer properties. Several population studies have suggested a link between increased garlic intake and reduced risk of certain cancers, including stomach and colorectal cancers. However, garlic supplements haven't been found to provide the same benefits, so skip the supplements and cook with garlic several times a week instead.

Selection: Choose firm garlic heads with the papery skin completely intact and without soft spots or sprouting. If it sprouts after you buy it, it's still okay to eat, but will just be less pungent.

Storage: Fresh garlic can be stored for one to two months. If you will use it relatively quickly, wrap it in netting or an open paper bag and store on the countertop, away from heat-generating appliances. Or, store it in a garlic keeper—a little pot that blocks light but has holes to allow air circulation. If you're not going to use your garlic right away, consider refrigerating it. Garlic will not only stay fresher longer in the refrigerator, its pungency and allicin content can also increase tenfold. Place it on a shelf in your refrigerator, not in the crisper drawer.

Preparation: Always chop, mince, slice, or crush garlic ten minutes before you eat it raw or expose it to the heat of cooking. During this time, the maximum amount of allicin is created, and it becomes heat-resistant, so the health-promoting properties of garlic are maximized and won't be destroyed in the heat. If you throw garlic into a hot pot without letting it rest first, its health-promoting properties will be destroyed in the heat.

Garlic skin should be papery and intact.

Avoid soft spots and sprouting.

❗ Expert Tip

To get rid of the garlic smell on your fingers after you chop a clove or two, run your fingers along your stainless steel sink or the flat edge of a stainless steel knife for thirty seconds. To get rid of garlic breath, chew a sprig of parsley.

GINGER

Ginger adds zing to just about any dish, and its unique, slightly spicy kick is an integral part of many Asian recipes and fresh juice blends. Healthwise, it offers powerful anti-inflammatory benefits and, therefore, may be helpful for those with inflammatory conditions such as acne or arthritis. It's traditionally used to soothe digestive upset and is well known for its ability to relieve gas. It can also help fight colds and flu by supporting the immune system and providing antiviral benefits.

Selection: You'll usually find ginger in the refrigerated area of the produce section. Choose ginger that's firm, smooth, and free of mold.

Storage: Refrigerate in the crisper drawer in a closed plastic bag with the air expelled.

Preparation: A little ginger goes a long way! Cut a half-inch to one-inch (1 to 2.5 cm) piece from the root and use the side of a spoon to peel off its skin easily. If you choose organic, there's no need to peel it for juices or blended preparations. Throw the whole piece into a juicer or blender for a smoothie or slice and dice it for a stir-fry. You could also make an after-dinner infusion: Place two to three thin slices of ginger at the bottom of a mug and then top with hot water. Ginger pairs very well with garlic, and together, they pack quite a medicinal punch!

Check for and avoid moldy pieces.

Ginger should feel firm.

GRAPEFRUIT

Grapefruit is an excellent source of vitamin C (one medium-size grapefruit contains more than 100 percent of your DV). This tart and tangy citrus fruit is often used in cleansing and fat-burning regimens as at least one study has found that eating half a fresh grapefruit daily promotes weight loss and improves insulin resistance. The ruby red or pink flesh is an indicator of its lycopene content, a phytonutrient that plays a role in protecting the skin from UV rays and cancer.

Small surface scratches are okay but avoid grapefruit with soft spots.

Selection: The fruit should feel heavy for its size and should be firm yet slightly springy when gentle pressure is applied. Grapefruits stored at room temperature should have a slightly sweet aroma. The color doesn't have to be perfect, and scratches and small surface imperfections shouldn't affect quality. Avoid any with an overly soft spot at the stem or with overly rough or wrinkled skin.

Storage: Store grapefruit at room temperature if consuming within a week of purchase. Otherwise, refrigerate in the crisper drawer where it'll last an additional week or two.

Preparation: Slice in half and then dig in with a spoon; juice them; or add them to smoothies.

Fruit should be firm with a slight spring to the touch.

GRAPES

Red and green grapes deliver a sweet-tart flavor in a perfect bite-size package, making them a fun, handy snack. Thanks to the wine industry's avid promotion, they're probably best known for their resveratrol content, a phytonutrient that plays a role in healthy aging and longevity. However, grapes have been found to contain more than 1,600 phytonutrients—and that's only what scientists have identified so far! Grape polyphenols—which, like resveratrol, are found in grapes of every color—support cell health and function, enhance cardiac health, and may also play a role in healthy aging.

Selection: Always choose organic grapes, as they routinely show up on the EWG's Dirty Dozen list. Grapes should still be attached to the vine and should look plump. Avoid any that look shriveled or are lighter in color near the stem. Grapes are available in green/white (which have a medium sweetness level), red/purple (which are very sweet), and blue/black (which are the least sweet). In general, the darker the color, the more phytonutrients it contains. Grapes may be seeded or seedless—the seeds are edible, however, and jut need to be chewed well.

Storage: Always refrigerate grapes. Wrap them in a paper towel in a closed plastic bag (like the one they're packaged in), and they should last up to five days.

Preparation: Wash your grapes and then pop them straight into your mouth! You can also freeze them for a super-refreshing treat or use them to top fruit or vegetable salads.

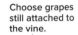

Choose grapes still attached to the vine.

Avoid grapes that are lighter in color near the stem.

GREENS

KALE, SPINACH, ARUGULA, SWISS CHARD, COLLARD GREENS & WATERCRESS

Dark leafy greens are like nature's multivitamins—loaded with an abundance of vitamins and minerals. For example, just one cup (67 g) of curly kale contains 133 percent DV of vitamin A, 134 percent DV of vitamin C, 10 percent DV of calcium, 7 percent DV of magnesium, and 6 percent DV of iron—and many other nutrients, too.

That same amount of kale clocks in at only 33 calories, but boasts 2 grams of protein and 5 percent DV of fiber. Because a meal-size salad usually contains about three to four cups (weights will vary) of greens, it's easy to see that simply adding greens to your diet packs a huge nutritional punch. Studies also show that greens help reduce cholesterol, aid in the body's natural detoxification process, protect against cancer, and support healthy bones thanks to their calcium, magnesium, and vitamin K content. (Note that spinach and beet greens generally provide less calcium than other greens because they contain oxalates, which block absorption.)

Leaves should be firm and crisp, not wilted or rubbery.

Selection: Choose organic greens to avoid pesticide exposure, as conventional varieties tend to be heavily sprayed. Spinach ranks as the seventh most heavily sprayed crop on the EWG's Dirty Dozen list, and conventional kale and collard greens are routinely sprayed with organophosphates, highly toxic chemicals that have been linked to leukemia, lymphoma, Parkinson's disease, decreased male fertility, and impaired intelligence and brain development in children. Choose organic kale and collard greens to avoid this toxic pesticide residue.

Look for leaves that feel firm and crisp and skip bunches that are wilted, rubbery, or yellow.

Storage: Kale should be stored in the crisper drawer of your refrigerator in either an open plastic bag (such as the one it's packaged in) or a micro-perforated bag (see page 56).

If you don't expect to eat the greens within the next two days, consider soaking and drying them as soon as you get home from the store. This process, as outlined by Jo Robinson in *Eating on the Wild Side*, takes about ten minutes but results in greens that last days longer than they would otherwise. To do this, submerge the greens in a bowl of cold water and soak for two to three minutes, swirling occasionally, to dislodge dirt, bugs, and debris. Lift the leaves out of the water into a strainer and then dump the water down the drain. (If you dump the leaves directly into the strainer, you'll be dumping debris back onto them.) Repeat two to three times until the water is clear. The cold water increases the greens' internal moisture and slows the aging process of the leaves, prolonging freshness. Dry with a salad spinner or towel to remove as much water as possible. Storing wet greens results in faster decay. Finally, put the greens in a resealable plastic bag, squeeze out as much air as possible without crushing the leaves, seal the bag, and use a pin to prick evenly spaced holes in the bag (ten holes for a quart, or 946 ml, bag and twenty holes for anything larger). Store in your refrigerator's crisper drawer.

Preparation: Greens can be eaten raw or cooked. If you're just starting to introduce greens into your diet, try them cooked first. The simplest method is to chop or chiffonade them, sauté with garlic and olive oil, and finish with a pinch of salt and, perhaps, some red pepper flakes.

For curly kale, the stem is edible but it's tough, so it's best removed. This is easy to do: Run your thumb and forefinger down the stem and gently pull off the leaves. You can also fold the leaf in half, flat, and then cut the stem out.

As for chard, its stems are softer and more pleasant to eat. Chop the stems and add them to the sauté pan along with the garlic, allowing them to cook for a minute or two before you add the leaves.

You can also braise or roast kale, chard, or collard greens with garlic and olive oil as a side dish—or make it a meal by adding chickpeas and sweet potatoes.

Use large collard or chard leaves as wraps, instead of tortillas. Baby spinach makes a delicious base for a salad and so does raw kale (with the right recipe, that is—if not marinated or massaged before serving, raw kale can be tough to chew).

Avoid greens that have become slimy.

81

BABY
SPINACH

COLLARD
GREENS

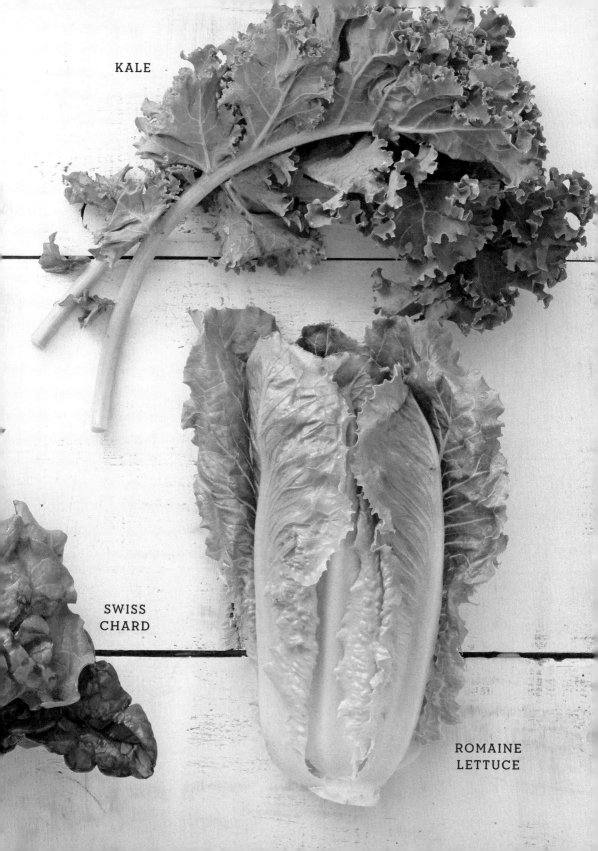

KALE

SWISS
CHARD

ROMAINE
LETTUCE

HERBS

Herbs add vibrant, distinct flavors to any dish and deliver plenty of antioxidants, nutrients, and health benefits. Even the most common herbs may help protect against diabetes, cancer, and heart disease.

Selection: When buying fresh herbs, choose bunches with green leaves that smell fresh. Avoid bunches that are wilted, have brown spots or yellow leaves, or feel slimy.

Storage: Increase the shelf life of soft herbs (including parsley, cilantro, dill, mint, and tarragon) by snipping the stems and putting them in a glass of water, as you would flowers, and then loosely placing a plastic bag (such as the one they came in) over the top and securing it with a rubber band. Apart from basil and very thin-leafed mint, all herbs should be refrigerated this way. Basil and thin-leafed mint should be stored in water on the countertop, away from light. (Try to change the water daily.) Herbs stored this way can last up to a week.

For sturdier herbs, such as rosemary, oregano, marjoram, and thyme: Wrap them first in a damp paper towel, then loosely in plastic wrap (or place in a zip-top bag or airtight container), and store in the crisper drawer of the refrigerator.

Choose herbs that stand upright and are not limp or slimy.

Preparation: Use herbs in salads, sauces, dressings, soups, drinks, smoothies, or anywhere else you'd like to add a hit of fresh flavor. For most dishes, use just the leaves, but for any blended preparations, throw the whole stalk in.

Basil

Fragrant basil is a powerful anti-inflammatory and antimicrobial. It contains a variety of nutrients that support cardiovascular health. Use it in pesto, add it to salads, or use as the finishing touch to any veggie, grain, or fish dish.

Cilantro

Cilantro has been found to exhibit powerful antibiotic activity, balance blood sugar, and aid in lowering cholesterol. Use cilantro in guacamole, salads, to top fish, or in Mexican and Asian dishes.

Mint

Prized for its ability to soothe the stomach, mint exhibits antibiotic activity, too. Muddle it in the bottom of a glass for a refreshing addition to water or lemonade or pour hot water over the leaves for an after-dinner digestive tea.

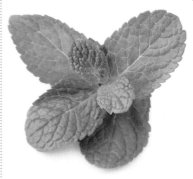

Oregano

Oregano is a medicinal herb, and though it's more widely used dried as a spice, you can sometimes find it fresh, too. Oregano contains a plethora of antioxidant compounds and is noted for its antibacterial, antiviral, and antifungal properties. Add it to sauces, soups, dressings, sautés, or any type of savory dish.

Avoid bunches of herbs that have brown spots or yellow leaves.

Parsley

Parsley adds fresh flavor to just about any dish. It is antioxidant rich and an excellent source of vitamins C and K. Use flat leaf parsley on fish and in salads. Curly parsley is generally reserved for use as a garnish.

Rosemary

A single whiff of rosemary is enough to enhance cognition and memory and reduce stress levels. It provides powerful antioxidants and has been shown to protect against bacteria, viruses, and cancer. Use it with grilled meat to counteract grilling's carcinogenic effects. Place a sprig of rosemary in or on whatever you're cooking to impart its fragrant flavor and then remove it before serving.

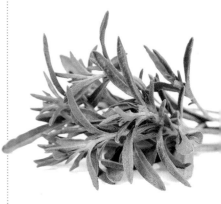

Tarragon

A staple of French cooking, tarragon imparts an anise-like flavor and aroma. It's rich in antioxidants and aids digestion. Use it raw in salads or mix it with other fresh herbs in a relish for fish.

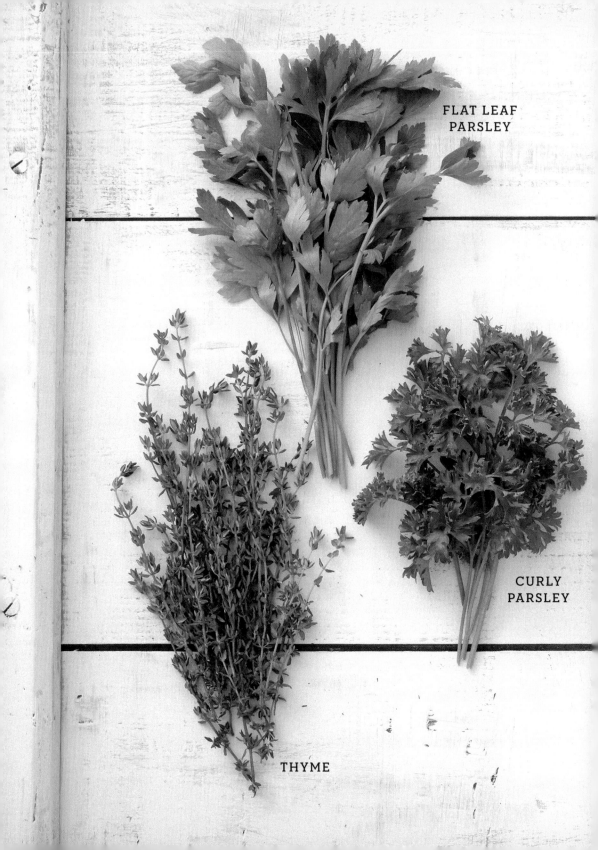

FLAT LEAF
PARSLEY

CURLY
PARSLEY

THYME

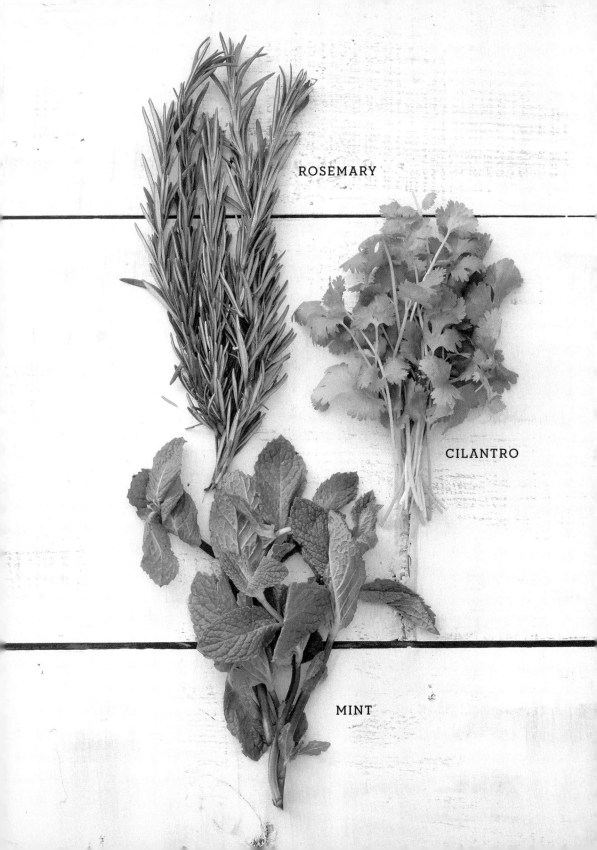

ROSEMARY

CILANTRO

MINT

HONEYDEW MELON

Honeydew is a juicy green melon that's about 90 percent water. It's an excellent source of a variety of antioxidants and vitamin C (delivering 51 percent DV per cup, or 170 g), which supports youthful-looking skin.

Selection: When buying whole honeydew, look for melons that feel heavy for their size and have no dents, fissures, or mold. The stem end of the fruit should have a slight depression, and it should smell sweet, like honeydew. If it has a stub, it was probably picked too soon and won't ripen and develop its flavor correctly.

When buying precut melon, choose those with the deepest green flesh. Avoid melon that has released a lot of liquid into the container, which is a sign it's not as fresh.

Storage: Honeydew will continue to ripen on the countertop. A ripe melon will last up to five days in the refrigerator's crisper drawer. Once cut, keep the seeds intact to help maintain freshness, cover with plastic wrap, and refrigerate for up to three days.

Preparation: Even though you won't be eating the rind, rinse honeydew well before cutting to remove any dirt or potentially harmful bacteria that could be transferred by a knife from the outside to the inside. To eat it, cut it in half, scoop out the seeds and pulp, and eat it with a spoon or cut it into wedges or cubes. Instead of slicing up the halves, you could fill the center with berries and coconut cream for an antioxidant-rich breakfast. Or, try blending a honeydew melon with basil for a refreshing summer smoothie.

The stem end will smell sweet when ripe.

Stem end should have a slight depression, not a stub, as shown here.

JICAMA

Jicama is a round root native to Mexico. Inside is a crisp, refreshing white flesh that tastes like a cross between a firm cucumber and a pear. It's high in fiber (6 grams per cup, or 130 g, for 24 percent DV) and low in calories (46 per cup, or 130 g), making it an excellent snack food or crunchy salad topping. If you're looking to lose weight, eat jicama regularly: It contains a type of prebiotic fiber that supports healthy digestion, weight control, and metabolic function.

Selection: Choose firm, fresh, thin-skinned jicama that's free from cracks, bruises, blemishes, mold, soft spots, and discoloration. Choose bulbs of less than 4 pounds (1.8 kg). These tend to be crisper and sweeter than larger ones.

Storage: Store jicama at room temperature or in the refrigerator for two to three weeks. Be sure to keep it dry as it will mold quickly if wet.

Preparation: Always peel and discard the inedible skin. Slice jicama into sticks for dipping in guacamole or other healthy dips. Cube it to add a little crunch to a salad or marinate the cubes in lime juice and chili powder for a snack or side dish. Grate or spiralize it for a softer texture or use a mandoline to thinly slice it and use the slices to make raw ravioli or mini taco wraps.

Avoid bruises, mold, or discoloration.

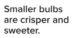

Smaller bulbs are crisper and sweeter.

LEEK

Leeks belong to the same family of vegetables as onions and garlic, called alliums. They're rich in sulfur-containing phytonutrients, although most of these nutrients are concentrated in the leaves and green portions of the stalk. They're completely edible, so eat these parts, too, instead of throwing them out! Leeks are also noted for their high levels of kaempferol, a phytochemical that may provide cardio-protective and cancer-protective benefits.

Selection: Leeks should be firm and straight, with white bulbs and dark green leaves. Buy the smallest leeks you can find because their leaves are more tender.

Storage: Refrigerate and eat leeks as soon as possible—ideally within three days because they lose their nutrient value quickly after harvest.

Preparation: Add sliced leeks to a stir-fry, an omelet, or a frittata. Braise it and serve it over fish or blend it into soups. You can even slice it thin and eat it raw in a salad. Again, be sure to use the nutrient-rich leaves and green portions, too!

Buy the smallest leeks you can find.

Leeks should be firm and straight, not bent or wilted.

LEMON & LIME

Lemons and limes do more than just preserve and flavor foods. They're a rich source of vitamin C (providing about 31 percent DV per quarter cup, or 60 ml, of juice), are bursting with antioxidants, and exhibit antibiotic effects. Perhaps the most interesting aspect of lemons and limes, though, is they are a source of limonids, which have been shown to help fight cancers of the mouth, skin, lung, breast, stomach, and colon in laboratory tests with animals and with human cells.

According to USDA research, they can remain in the bloodstream for up to twenty-four hours in some people, which may help explain their anticancer effects. It's also significant because similar anticarcinogens don't remain in the bloodstream for nearly as long. Phenols in green tea or dark chocolate, for instance, only remain active in the body for four to six hours.

Selection: Lemons and limes should be firm but not hard and should have glossy skin without soft spots. The juiciest fruits are heavy for their size. Lemons should be a deep yellow color with no hint of green. For limes, look for the lightest green, almost yellowish, fruit as these will be ripest. The peels have more antioxidants than the juice or flesh so buy organic and eat the zest, too.

Storage: Lemons and limes will last at room temperature for about a week. They'll keep an additional week in the refrigerator. If you're not going to use them within that timeframe, squeeze the juice and freeze it.

Preparation: Squeeze lemon juice into hot water and sip first thing in the morning for a cleansing, energizing start to your day. You can also steep the peels (just make sure they're organic). Use lemon juice instead of vinegar in dressings or on salads or squeeze it over fish. Use the zest in pies, breads, cakes, sauces, and salad dressings. You can also use it to top steamed vegetables.

Lemons and limes should feel firm, not hard.

Skin should be glossy without soft spots.

LETTUCE

Until dark leafy greens stole the spotlight, lettuce was the standard salad base. While lettuce may be less nutrient dense than the more popular kale and arugula, its many varieties still offer plenty of benefits, notably fiber, vitamins A, C, and K, calcium, iron, and even a little protein.

Selection: Ideally, choose organic lettuce as it's one of the more heavily sprayed crops (ranked number seventeen out of fifty items on the EWG's 2015 *Shopper's Guide to Pesticides in Produce*). Look for leaves that feel firm and crisp and ignore bunches that are wilted, rubbery, or yellow.

Most nutritious varieties: Red leaf, green leaf, romaine, radicchio, endive, escarole, frisée, mizuna, watercress, tatsoi, Bibb, and butter

Least nutritious varieties: Iceberg

Storage: If you plan to consume your lettuce within two days of purchasing it, you can usually get away with storing it in an open plastic bag in your refrigerator's crisper drawer. Just wrap the lettuce in a piece of paper towel to absorb any excess moisture (from ice or water mist from market displays) and then place it back in the plastic bag.

To store it for longer, wash it using the same method detailed for Greens (pages 80–81).

Preparation: Remove the stem and either tear or cut it into bite-size pieces for a salad. Certain varieties, such as radicchio, endive, or romaine, are great for use as a cup or wrap to hold other ingredients. To reap the benefits of the fat-soluble vitamins, such as vitamins A and K, always eat lettuce with some sort of fat, such as oil, nuts, seeds, or avocado.

Avoid bunches that look wilted or yellow.

Buy organic.

MANGO

It may be hard to believe that mangos, with their super-sweet flesh, are not only bursting with nutrients, but low glycemic, too. Just one cup (175 g) provides 100 percent DV of vitamin C, 12 percent DV of fiber, and 35 percent DV of vitamin A.

Selection: The best indicator of ripeness is scent, not color. The stem area will smell like mango when it's ripe. If it smells like ammonia, it's a sign that the fruit is past its prime. Firmness is another indicator. When squeezed gently, the fruit should give slightly. If it's too soft and almost mushy, it's past its prime. If it's too firm, it needs time to ripen, so leave it on the countertop to do so.

Storage: If you plan to eat a mango soon after purchase or if it needs to ripen, store it on the countertop. Ripe mangos should be stored in your refrigerator's crisper drawer and will only last two to three days.

Preparation: There is a wide, thin, center pit in a mango, but it's easy to cut around. Lay the mango on a cutting board with the stem facing away from you and cut about one-quarter inch (6 mm) to the left of center and then about one-quarter inch (6 mm) to the right of center. You'll end up with two halves. Score them into strips or cubes and then use a spoon to scoop out the flesh. You can eat mango on its own; add it to smoothies; freeze it and then throw it in the blender to make sorbet; or add it to dessert recipes, such as mango sticky rice.

Scent is the best indicator of ripeness, not color.

Avoid fruit that feels soft rather than firm.

MUSHROOM

WHITE BUTTON, CREMINI, PORTABELLO, SHIITAKE, MAITAKE & OYSTER

Pale in color and covered in dirt, mushrooms may not look like much at first glance. But in Asia, they're considered a symbol of health and longevity and are widely used in traditional Chinese medicine thanks to their immune-boosting properties. They are suprisingly antioxidant-rich and studies indicate regular consumption may help protect against cardiovascular disease.

From the humble white button to the exotic shiitake mushroom, pile them on for good health. They're also a great weight-loss food, as they're low in calories, moderate in fiber, and highly filling. An entire cup (121 g) of grilled portobello mushrooms contains only forty-two calories, yet offers 11 percent DV of fiber and five grams of protein.

Selection: Choose organic because mushrooms absorb much of the pollutants in the air, water, and soil in which they grow. Find caps that are smooth and unblemished and avoid slimy ones. For small button mushrooms, flip them over: If the cap is separating from the stem, the mushroom is less fresh. Instead, choose ones with no gap between cap and stem.

Most nutritious varieties: shiitake, maitake

Storage: Never store mushrooms in a plastic bag or in an open container, both of which speed their demise. Instead, refrigerate them in a closed paper bag and they'll last about a week.

Preparation: To clean mushrooms, wipe them with a damp paper towel to remove all the dirt. You can add sliced mushrooms to the pot when cooking brown rice or other grains to impart an earthy flavor. Raw mushrooms contain compounds that interfere with the absorption of nutrients, so always eat them cooked.

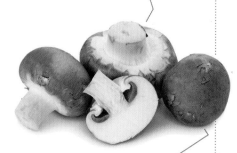

For button mushrooms, there should be no gaps or tears between the caps and stems.

Caps should be smooth, not sticky or slimy.

OKRA

A staple in Indian, African, and Middle Eastern cuisines, okra tends to be overlooked in the United States—and that's unfortunate, considering its health benefits. Okra contains mucilage, which balances blood sugar, reduces cholesterol, and helps sweep the digestive tract and seed it with good bacteria. It may also reduce digestive issues, such as gas and bloating. When sliced, okra looks like little stars, adding a fun crunch to salads or sautéed veggie dishes.

Selection: Choose small, slender, firm green pods, avoiding the ones specked with purple or black.

Storage: Store in your refrigerator's crisper drawer.

Preparation: Discard the stem and slice the remaining pod into quarter-inch (6 mm) pieces. Use raw in salads; lightly stir-fry; or look up traditional ethnic recipes, such as India's *bhindi masala* or Ethiopia's *bamya alich'a*. If you're new to okra, it's probably best to lightly stir-fry it or use it in one of these traditional recipes to become acquainted with its unique taste and texture before trying it raw.

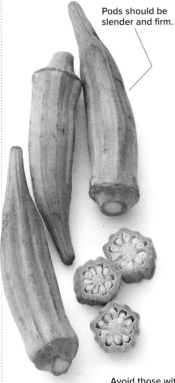

Pods should be slender and firm.

Avoid those with black or purple spots.

ONIONS, SHALLOTS & SCALLIONS

The humble onion is packed with health benefits. Onions contain quercetin, a phytonutrient noted for its antibacterial, antiviral, and anticancer properties.

Shallots are milder than onions but contain twice as much quercetin. Scallions, or green onions, are another highly nutritious yet milder pick, with hundreds of phytonutrients.

Selection: Choose small onions that are firm to the touch with skin that's intact and free of soft spots. For shallots, look for firm ones with tight outer skin and no bruising or soft spots. For scallions, look for those with crisp, green tops and a firm white base. They should not be slimy.

Most nutritious varieties: Red, purple, Western Yellow, and New York Bold onions, shallots, and scallions

Least nutritious varieties: Vidalia, Western White, and Empire Sweet onions

Storage: Store onions and shallots on the countertop in an open bowl, a net bag, or open paper bag. To store them for longer than two weeks, refrigerate and they will last up to a month. Store scallions with their roots still attached in a small glass of water on the countertop or in the fridge. If you cut off the top green portion, they will continue to grow—just remember to change the water daily. (The new shoots will be milder.) They also can be stored in a micro-perforated bag (see page 56), but are best eaten within a few days.

Preparation: Eat onions, shallots, and scallions raw or cooked. Use shallots in any recipe in which you'd use onions; they're just slightly milder. Use the entire scallion—both white and green parts.

The outer skin should be intact.

Red and purple varieties have more antioxidants.

ORANGE

Oranges are well known for their high vitamin C content (providing 93 percent DV per orange), which supports immunity, prevents free radical damage, and encourages youthful-looking skin. Oranges contain more than 170 different phytonutrients, providing powerful antioxidant protection and anti-inflammatory benefits. They're even a good source of limonids, the powerful anticancer phytonutrients also found in lemons.

Selection: When selecting an organic orange, it's simple: Choose the orange that's the deepest shade of orange.

When it comes to conventional oranges, though, be aware of this trick. Conventional oranges may have been "degreened": That is, they may have been picked when underripe and then exposed to ethylene gas in a warehouse to quickly turn the skin orange so the fruit appears ripe in the store. However, the gas has no effect on the flesh inside, so the orange will still be sour. When choosing conventional oranges that are all the same color, choose the larger fruits—this indicates they remained on the tree for longer and are probably riper. If your supermarket display features oranges in a variety of shades, then they weren't degreened—in which case, choose the most orange orange.

Most nutritious varieties: Blood oranges, Cara Cara, and navel

Storage: Eat oranges within a few days of purchase or remove them from their plastic bag and store on a shelf or in the crisper drawer of the refrigerator.

Preparation: Enjoy ripe oranges on their own or use in salads, sauces, or dressings. The most nutritious part of an orange is the white pith, so be sure to include it when blending into smoothies or sauces.

For organic oranges, choose those that are the deepest in color.

For non-organic, choose the largest size fruits.

PAPAYA

Sweet, creamy papaya brings the taste of the tropics home and is an excellent source of vitamin C (144 percent DV per cup, or 140 g), vitamin A (31 percent DV), folate (13 percent DV), and fiber (10 percent DV). Vitamins A and C are powerful antioxidants, which may help protect against disease and keep skin clear and youthful. Papaya contains an enzyme called papain, which can help decrease inflammation and may support digestive health.

Selection: Color is the most important indicator of ripeness. Ripe papaya is mostly yellow or orange-yellow. The body of the fruit should give slightly when pressed, while the neck or stem area should be firm, not soft. Papaya will ripen on the countertop. A semi-ripe papaya that's equal parts yellow and green should ripen in two to four days. Don't worry about brown freckles on the skin—they don't detract from the flavor.

Most nutritious varieties: To avoid GMOs, buy organic papaya or those grown in Mexico or Belize, including varieties such as Mexican Red, Caribbean Red, Maradol, Royal Star, Singapore Pink, and Higgins.

Least nutritious varieties: Certain varieties, typically those produced in Hawaii, are genetically modified (GMO), including Rainbow, Sunrise, and Sunup Strawberry varieties.

Storage: Store on the countertop and eat within a week.

Preparation: Slice in half, discard the seeds, and scoop out the flesh to eat on its own or add to smoothies. (Papaya seeds are edible, although unpleasant, and have been traditionally used medicinally.) Fill papaya halves with coconut ice cream or berries or cube papaya and drizzle with lime juice and chili powder. Green (unripe) papaya can be sliced and used in traditional Asian salads.

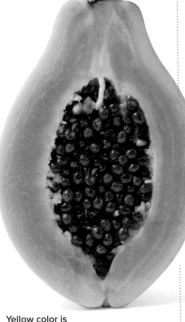

The neck or stem should be firm, not soft.

Yellow color is the most important indicator of ripeness.

PARSNIP

Parsnips are often overlooked in the grocery store, but these sweet root vegetables, which look like white carrots, are as pleasing to the palate as they are to the waistline. They taste sweet just like carrots, and are best when roasted to bring out their caramelized flavor. They contain just 100 calories per cup (110 g), plus a whopping 7 grams (or 36 percent DV) of fiber. They're also loaded with nutrients, providing more than 20 percent of the recommended DV for folate, vitamin C, vitamin K, and manganese.

Selection: Parsnips are off-white in color and typically have traces of dirt. Choose thinner parsnips to ensure they're sweet and tender; larger, thicker parsnips have an unpleasant, thick, woody core. Ideally, choose parsnips with greens and roots intact and avoid any that are shriveled, yellowing, or browning at the top near the stem.

Storage: Refrigerate in a sealed plastic bag in the crisper drawer where they'll last up to two weeks.

Preparation: Parsnips are best when roasted because roasting enhances their sweetness. Eat roasted parsnips on their own, blend into soups, or purée into a side dish that's similar to mashed potatoes. They're also tasty grated raw into salads.

Avoid browning, yellowing, or shriveling near the stem.

Thin parsnips are sweet and tender.

PEAR

Tart and slightly sweet, pears are a high-fiber fruit—just one pear provides 22 percent of your recommended daily intake. That means they make a filling, satisfying snack or addition to breakfast, particularly when dipped in nut butter or paired with a handful of nuts. Be sure to eat the skin, as research indicates about half of a pear's fiber is retained there. Plus, the skin has three to four times the amount of certain phytonutrients in comparison to the flesh.

Selection: Pears are highly perishable when ripe, so most grocery stores sell unripe pears, which will ripen in a day or two on your countertop. Pears should be firm to the touch, but not too hard. They should have smooth skin that's free of bruises. To test for ripeness, instead of squeezing the whole fruit, pinch it near the top toward the stem. If it's slightly soft, it's ripe enough to eat.

Storage: Store unripe pears on the countertop and consume soon after they ripen. To preserve ripe pears longer, refrigerate them where they'll last a few extra days.

Preparation: Eat pears on their own as a snack; dice them into oatmeal or add to smoothies; slice them and spread with almond butter; or bake and sprinkle with cinnamon for a healthy dessert.

To test ripeness, pinch near the top of the stem to see if slightly soft.

Look for smooth skin that is free of bruises.

PEPPER, BELL

Crisp, refreshing bell peppers come in a rainbow of colors, from red, orange, and yellow to green, purple, and black. Plenty of nutrients accompany those bright colors, too, including vitamins C, A, and B_6 as well as a number of anti-inflammatory antioxidants, such as lutein and zea-xanthin, which are both crucial to eye health as well as quercetin, which may play a role in reducing stress and supporting cardiovascular health.

Selection: Always choose organic as peppers clock in at number ten on the EWG's 2016 Dirty Dozen list. Choose peppers with smooth vibrantly colored skin, free of wrin-kling, dimpling, or soft spots. They should be firm and heavy for their size, indicating thick, well-hydrated walls, and the stems should be green and look fresh.

Storage: Store bell peppers in an open plastic bag in your refrigerator's crisper drawer where they'll last for seven to ten days. If you're not going to eat them within a few days, you may want to add a damp paper towel to the bag to help them retain moisture.

Preparation: Bell peppers add a lovely crunch to salads and are delicious sautéed with onions, too. Add them to a veggie stir-fry—or try slicing and eating them raw, dipped in hummus or tapenade.

Stems should be green and fresh looking, not brown.

Skin should not be wrinkled or dimpled.

PEPPER, HOT
JALAPEÑO, SERRANO & CHILE

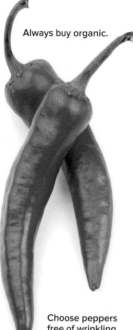

Always buy organic.

Choose peppers free of wrinkling, dimpling, or soft spots.

Hot peppers don't just add a kick to your meals, they may also help whittle your waistline. They contain capsaicin, a compound that might promote weight loss—especially of hard-to-lose belly fat—by increasing energy expenditure after consumption. Plus, hot peppers provide anti-inflammatory benefits and promote healthy blood flow.

Selection: Always choose organic hot peppers as they routinely end up on the EWG's Dirty Dozen list (page 46)—not for having the largest number of pesticides, but for being sprayed with the most toxic ones. Data from the USDA in 2010 and 2011 found three toxic insecticides on some hot peppers in concentrations high enough to cause concern.

Choose peppers with vibrantly colored smooth skin, free of wrinkling, dimpling, or soft spots. Striations, though, don't affect quality and may indicate a higher nutrient value. Peppers should be firm and feel heavy for their size. Jalapeños start off green and get milder—and turn red—as they mature. Serranos, a more slender green pepper and another staple of Mexican cuisine, are hotter than jalapeños. Habanero peppers are short and squat, come in a variety of oranges, reds, and yellows, and are usually the hottest variety of pepper available at the grocery store.

Storage: Store in a plastic bag with a damp paper towel in your refrigerator's crisper drawer where they should last seven to ten days.

Preparation: The hottest part of hot peppers is the seeds and the white pith inside, so adjust the heat of your dishes by using less or more of these. Add chopped or sliced peppers to a stir-fry, omelets, chili, salsa, guacamole, or just about any dish that needs a little kick!

PINEAPPLE

Sweet, juicy pineapple is an excellent source of vitamin C, which supports youthful-looking skin and a healthy immune system (one cup, or 165 g, provides more than 100 percent of your daily recommended intake). Apart from its tropical taste, pineapple may be best known for its bromelain content, an enzyme that supports healthy digestion. The fruit also provides a hefty dose of manganese (77 percent DV per cup, or 165 g), a mineral in which an estimated 37 percent of Americans are deficient. (Some studies suggest that adequate manganese may ease PMS symptoms.) Plus, as it provides 9 percent of the recommended daily intake of fiber per cup (165 g), pineapple makes a filling snack or satisfying addition to smoothies.

Selection: Look for pineapples that are heavy for their size and free from soft spots or darkened "eyes." The crown leaves should be dark green with no signs of fading or browning. Try to pluck a leaf from the crown. If one comes out, the fruit is past its prime.

Storage: Because pineapples are harvested when ripe, they don't keep well. Eat within one to two days or refrigerate for up to four days. When you leave a pineapple out at room temperature it becomes juicier and softer, so if you're storing yours in the fridge, you may want to take it out a day or two before you plan to serve it.

Preparation: Lay the pineapple on its side to chop off the crown and then stand it up and cut it into a cube by slicing straight down all four sides. (You may need to go back and slice off a little more skin at the corners.) The sides you remove contain a lot of juice: squeeze them into a glass for a shot of fresh juice. Then slice the peeled pineapple into rounds or cubes to eat. The center core is edible, but it's tough to chew. So before eating, remove it, but add it to the blender for extra fiber in smoothies. Pineapple is a good match for savory dishes—try it grilled, in a veggie stir-fry, or a curry dish.

Leaves should be dark green and not easily plucked.

"Eyes" should not be dark.

POMEGRANATE

Ruby red pomegranate arils (seeds) offer antioxidant-rich bursts of sweet-tart juice. Also known as a Chinese apple, this exotic fruit has become more readily available in American grocery stores, but you'll probably only find them between September and January because they have a short season. They're probably best known for their connection to heart health, as they've been found to reduce inflammation and help lower cholesterol and blood pressure.

Selection: Select pomegranates that are heavy for their size as they'll be the juiciest. Don't worry too much about the color of the rind. It's not an indicator of quality, and it may be bright red, reddish-brown, or anything in between. Avoid any with soft shriveled skin, bruises, or cracks. As their popularity increases, you may also find the arils in containers in the refrigerated section of the grocery store—a perfectly acceptable option.

Storage: Pomegranates should be kept on the countertop, although they'll last much longer when refrigerated—at least three to four weeks. Once they've been opened and seeded, the arils should be refrigerated or frozen in a tightly sealed bag.

Preparation: Score the skin of the pomegranate into four quarters and carefully pull apart the four pieces. In the sink, fill a large bowl with water and submerge the quarters. Use your fingers to gently rub the arils off (the water prevents the red juice from splattering everywhere). The arils will sink to the bottom, while the white membrane and skin will float to the top. Remove what is floating on top and then dump the arils into a colander. Eat as a snack on their own (I pour the arils into a bowl and eat them with a spoon); blend into smoothies; or use to top salads, roasted veggies, or oatmeal. They do have a center seed, which is edible—just chew them well!

Heavy fruit has the most juice.

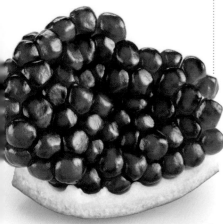

Color of the rind may be variable from bright red to reddish-brown.

POTATO

Potatoes get a bad rap: They're often demonized and labeled an indulgence. In fact, Harvard's Healthy Eating Plate doesn't count potatoes toward your vegetable servings as they have the same effect on blood sugar as refined grains and sweets. And though it's true that potatoes are no nutritional match for other veggies, such as kale, and many potato preparations—such as french fries, cheese fries, and potato chips—are even worse, certain types of potatoes do have nutritional merit. Though you don't need to eat potatoes as part of a healthy diet, choosing the right varieties and cooking techniques can make eating potatoes a guilt-free pleasure.

Selection: In general, choose firm potatoes with the darkest skins and flesh. Choose organic, as potatoes are one of the most heavily sprayed crops, ranking number fifteen on the EWG's *Shopper's Guide to Pesticides in Produce*.

Most nutritious varieties: Purple Peruvian potatoes are not only the most nutrient-dense variety, but they also add a vibrant pop of color to your plate. French fingerling, large purple, and Ozette fingerling also rank highly in terms of antioxidants. New potatoes, freshly harvested small potatoes with thin skin, such as small red or white potatoes or boiling potatoes, are a good, easy-to-find choice. (Sweet potatoes aren't actually potatoes: see their entry on page 110.)

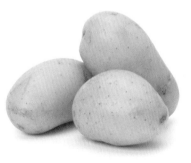

No matter the variety, potatoes should feel firm.

Least nutritious varieties: Old potatoes, such as Russet Burbank, Irish, and Yukon varieties, do contain a variety of vitamins and minerals, but are more higher glycemic than others. That said, try swapping them for lower-glycemic potatoes, listed previously, in your favorite recipes—or, if you're going to eat them, try the special preparation techniques that follow.

Storage: Due to their thin skins, new potatoes don't store well, so keep them refrigerated and eat within a week.

Old potatoes, also known as storage potatoes, are those harvested when fully mature and then cured for a few weeks to increase shelf life before they make it to the grocery store. If using these, store them in a cool dark place with good ventilation—for example, in a netted bag or open paper bag—where they can last for two to three months.

Preparation: The skin is the most nutrient-dense part of the potato, so choose organic and eat the skin. If you're cooking with nonorganic potatoes, peel the skin to avoid about 70 percent of the toxic chemicals with which they were sprayed. Some of the chemicals used are water soluble, so the other 30 percent typically remains inside the potato's flesh.

If using old potatoes, you can make them healthier by reducing their glycemic load. Just cook them and then refrigerate for twenty-four hours before eating. The cool temperature converts the rapidly digested starch into one that's more resistant—one that's broken down more slowly and is gentler on the body. This works well for any type of potato salad. Even if you reheat the chilled potatoes, they retain their lower glycemic status, and this simple chilling technique can reduce your blood sugar spike by as much as 25 percent.

Cook potatoes with fat or dress them in fat (such as olive oil) to slow digestion, thereby reducing their glycemic load (and your blood sugar spike). So, if you're baking or steaming them, be sure to dress them in olive oil afterward. Or, simply roast, sauté, or steam and dress with oil. (Still craving your old favorites? Instead of mashed potatoes, try mashed cauliflower. Instead of french fries, try baked sweet potato fries.)

ⓘ Expert Tip

High glycemic foods spike blood sugar more than others. A diet filled with high glycemic foods is associated with weight gain and diabetes, so it's best to consume a low glycemic diet for optimum health.

Choose those with the darkest skins for added nutrients.

RADISH

Crisp, crunchy, and slightly spicy, radishes are heavy on health benefits—living proof that good things come in small packages. As a member of the cruciferous vegetable family, they contain glucosinolates, highly regarded for their anticancer potential. In traditional Chinese medicine and Ayurvedic medicine, radishes are revered for their ability to break down and expel toxins and mucus, so they're often used in sore throat remedies and digestive system cleanses. In fact, there's a proverb in traditional Chinese medicine that's similar to the Western saying, "An apple a day keeps the doctor away." It goes, "Eat white radish in the winter and ginger in the summer, and you won't need to trouble the doctor for a prescription."

Selection: Choose radishes that are firm and unblemished, with their bright green leaves still attached. Avoid any with slimy leaves or a strong smell. When in season, try beautiful watermelon radishes, French breakfast radishes, or the long white daikon radish.

Storage: Remove the greens from the radishes and store them in a plastic bag in your refrigerator's crisper drawer. They'll last about three to five days.

Preparation: Slice radishes and eat raw as crudités with a healthy dip, such as tapenade or hummus; grate or slice into a salad; or top your avocado toast with a few thin slices for extra crunch and flavor.

Radishes should be firm and unblemished.

Avoid radishes with a strong smell.

SALAD GREENS
IN A CLAMSHELL

Choosing salad greens in a plastic clamshell is a convenient way to buy them. Depending on the season, you'll find a mix of baby spinach, baby arugula, baby kale, mesclun, and various blends. They're typically triple washed and ready to eat. (Some sources still suggest washing them before eating.)

Selection: Conventionally-grown lettuce and greens typically undergo heavy pesticide spraying, so choose organic. Browse through the packages to find the one with the latest expiration date as this will be the freshest. Baby arugula, baby spinach, and baby kale are all top picks.

Storage: Store the clamshell in the refrigerator. If any leaves start to turn slimy, throw out the entire package. Slimy leaves are a sign that bacteria is growing, and it can easily spread, so don't consume it. (If it goes bad before the expiration date, most stores will happily replace it.) Also, pick out any yellow or brown speckled leaves, which are a sign they're past their prime.

Preparation: Use salad greens as a base for raw salads; in smoothies or omelets; or sauté baby spinach or baby kale as a side dish.

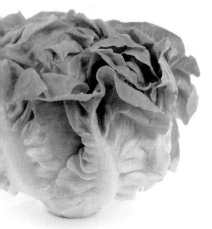

Avoid brown or yellow specked leaves.

Avoid anything that looks slimy.

SQUASH, WINTER
ACORN, BUTTERNUT & SPAGHETTI

Brightly colored winter squashes roast deliciously, providing nutrition and warmth during chilly fall and winter months.

Selection: With all squashes, choose those that feel heavy for their size and have firm flesh. The skin should be matte, not glossy. Glossy skin indicates the squash was picked too soon and won't be as sweet.

Storage: Stored in a cool, dry place (not the refrigerator) with plenty of ventilation, a whole winter squash should keep for up to three months. Cut pieces should be refrigerated and will last up to a week.

Preparation: Slice the squash in half, scoop out the seeds and pulp, and roast. It can then be used in soups or purées. You could also cut the flesh into cubes and then steam, sauté, or roast them.

Acorn Squash
Acorn squash is great when stuffed. It has a slightly sweet, nutty-tasting flesh that melts in your mouth when roasted. It contains small amounts of a wide variety of vitamins and minerals, including potassium, magnesium, and vitamin C.

Butternut Squash
Bright orange butternut squash may be sweet, but it's a great match for savory dishes, too. It's loaded with vitamins A and C, plus a variety of minerals, including potassium, magnesium, and manganese. It's best roasted or puréed into a soup.

Spaghetti Squash
It's fun to eat and simple to make! When you roast spaghetti squash, running a fork across its cooked flesh splits it into pasta-like strands that are low in calories and low glycemic. Use it to get your pasta fix—minus the calories.

Skin should be matte not glossy.

Choose those that feel heavy for their size.

SWEET POTATO

Sweet potatoes aren't potatoes, or yams, for that matter, although they are often mistakenly labeled as such in the grocery store.

The bright orange color of the flesh is an indicator of its high amount of vitamin A (nearly 400 percent of your DV per cup, or 133 g). Even though it's sweet, the sweet potato has a lower glycemic load than a white potato, which makes it a better choice than the pale-fleshed doppelgangers. Don't shy away from sweet potatoes! They're good for you.

Selection: Choose sweet potatoes that feel firm, don't have any bruising or soft spots, and have bright orange flesh. Because the skin is the most nutritious part, choose organic and eat it. If you can find purple sweet potatoes, grab them. Their fun color will brighten your plate, and they contain anthocyanins, an antioxidant being studied for its potentially potent anticancer properties. "Garnet" or "jewel" varieties are, in fact, sweet potatoes, not yams.

Storage: Sweet potatoes will last about a week at room temperature, but they'll last longer in a cool dark place in an unsealed paper bag. Don't refrigerate them because it changes their flavor and texture.

Preparation: Steam or roast sweet potatoes—both preparations double their antioxidant value. Don't boil them: It leaches the water-soluble vitamin A right out of them! The skin is more nutritious than the flesh, so choose organic and eat the whole thing.

Choose sweet potatoes that feel firm to the touch, not soft or spongy.

Flesh should be bright orange.

110

TOMATOES

Tomatoes are rich in a variety of antioxidants, including lycopene, believed to be a powerful protector against certain cancers, including those of the prostate, lung, and stomach.

If you're concerned about heart health, add more tomatoes to your diet. They are linked to a decreased risk of developing high blood pressure and heart disease because of their antioxidant support and regulation of fat in the blood, which helps lower "bad" LDL cholesterol.

Note that tomatoes belong to the nightshade family, so, if you have an inflammatory condition, consider avoiding them to see whether it brings any relief.

Selection: Look for plump, richly colored, firm, heavy tomatoes with smooth skin. Avoid those with bruises or soft spots, and choose organic, as they are routinely part of the EWG Dirty Dozen list.

Tomatoes taste best when in season. So head to the farmers' market and pick heirloom varieties, which are infinitely more flavorful than what you'll find at the grocery store.

Storage: Tomatoes stored in the fridge become mealy and less flavorful. Take them out of the plastic bag and store them on the countertop, away from direct sunlight. They will last up to a week, depending on how ripe they were when purchased.

The only exception is during the summer. If they are especially ripe and you want to extend their shelf life, the fridge will preserve them for another day or so. After removal, let them sit for 30 minutes on the counter to return to room temperature for best flavor and juiciness.

Preparation: Eat tomatoes raw or cooked. Cooking them increases the availability of lycopene, so cook them down into a sauce or soup or lightly stir-fry them before folding into an omelet. Pairing them with fat, such as olive oil, also increases availability. Slow-roast tomatoes in a 300°F (150°C, or gas mark 2) oven for two hours.

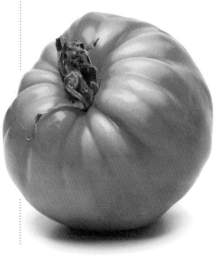

Heirloom varieties, such as the one below, are among the most flavorful.

WATERMELON

Tap the watermelon: it should sound hollow not flat.

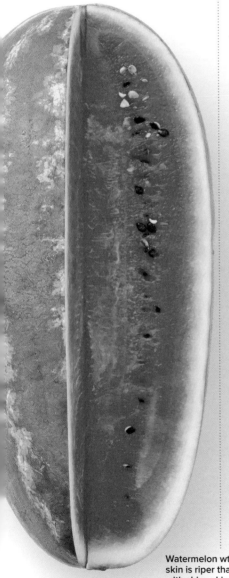

Watermelon with dull skin is riper than fruit with shiny skin.

Watermelon is 92 percent water, which means this juicy, summer melon makes a wonderfully hydrating breakfast or snack. It's an excellent source of lycopene, which supports cardiovascular health and may provide some sun protection when eaten regularly. It also supplies vitamins C and A, both of which promote glowing skin. What's the best part? Though many people avoid watermelon because it's "too sugary," the truth is that it has a surprisingly low glycemic load. That means it shouldn't cause a large blood sugar spike, so eat up!

Selection: A fully ripened watermelon should feel heavy for its size. The rind should be smooth yet dull; as it ripens it loses its shine. The "ground spot," or the flat side where the watermelon rested on the soil as it grew, should be creamy yellow in color. If it's white or green, the watermelon probably isn't fully ripe. Tapping the watermelon should produce a hollow sound rather than a flat thump.

If you can find watermelon with seeds, go for it—the seeds are edible, so you don't have to spit them out as you eat. Chew them well for added protein and minerals. They're a particularly good source of zinc.

If you prefer to buy precut watermelon, choose halves, quarters, or wedges with the reddest flesh. When the rind is attached in this way, it's likely that the slices were cut at the grocer's—while cubed, rind-free melon is usually cut at a faraway processing plant and is probably not as fresh.

Storage: Whole melons should be stored on the countertop. For a cold treat, refrigerate just before serving. Cut watermelon should always be refrigerated.

Preparation: Watermelon is best when sliced or cubed and eaten on its own. You can blend it to make watermelon water or a smoothie, chop it into salads, or purée it into a refreshing chilled gazpacho.

YAM

Though the term "yam" is often used interchangeably with "sweet potato," the truth is the two roots aren't even related to one another. Native to Africa, yams are starchier and are not commonly sold outside ethnic markets (regardless of the display sign at your local grocery!). They're not as sweet or as nutritious as sweet potatoes, but they still contain a variety of antioxidants, vitamins, and minerals.

Selection: True yams have a dark brown or black, bark-like skin and white, purple, or reddish flesh. They come in many varieties and can be as small as regular potatoes or upwards of five feet (150 cm) long. Select yams that feel firm and have unwrinkled flesh. Note that anything labeled "garnet" or "jewel" is actually a sweet potato, not a yam.

Storage: Store them in a cool, dark, dry place, but do not refrigerate.

Preparation: If you do find true yams, they should always be cooked, never eaten raw. Traditionally boiled, they retain more flavor when prepared by other cooking methods, such as baking. Wrap them in aluminum foil and bake in a 450°F (230°C, or gas mark 8) oven for about one hour until tender. Or, peel, dice, drizzle with olive oil, dust with spices, and roast until slightly caramelized.

Anything labeled "garnet" or "jewel" is actually a sweet potato, not a yam.

Look for firm, unwrinkled flesh.

YUCCA

Should look firm not shriveled.

Yucca, also known as cassava, is a root vegetable that tastes similar to potatoes, but is superior in health benefits and nutrition. Yucca contains nutrients that may help reduce blood pressure and high cholesterol. It's a good source of a variety of minerals, including potassium, manganese, and magnesium. It's also an excellent source of vitamin C (71 percent DV per cup, or 206 g). While you might not be familiar with whole yucca, you've probably already tasted it as tapioca, which is simply the starch extracted from it.

Selection: Choose firm roots that aren't shriveled. The inner flesh should be creamy white without any black or brown spots. Because yucca doesn't turn over quickly at most grocery stores—and as it goes bad quickly—ask the produce manager to cut it in half so you can check its freshness before buying. Only purchase what you'll use in the next day or two.

Storage: Store yucca on the countertop or in another cool, dry place, out of the sun. Aim to use it within two to three days of purchase.

Preparation: Yucca that's long and thin is easier to work with. Although the skin may look thick and tough, it's easy to peel with a vegetable peeler. Remove all the brown peel to reveal the white center. Cut it into three-inch-long (7.5 cm) pieces and boil for thirty minutes. Drain and let cool. Remove and discard the center vein and then chop it into bite-size pieces and season with garlic and oil. To make fries, after boiling, cut the yucca into french fry wedges. Coat them in oil and spices and bake for thirty minutes at 400°F (200°C, or gas mark 6), turning them halfway through.

Flesh should be creamy white and free of black or brown spots.

ZUCCHINI/ SUMMER SQUASH

Although not particularly vibrant in color, summer squash is still a great source of antioxidants, vitamins, and minerals. Of note, it's a source of lutein and zeaxanthin, two phytonutrients that support eye health. It also contains manganese and vitamin C, which provide a variety of benefits, including supporting cardiovascular health. If you're looking to lose weight, add zucchini to your diet. It's low in calories, low glycemic, and high in fiber (10 percent DV per cup, or 120 g), making it a filling, satisfying way to peel off the pounds.

Selection: Choose squash with unblemished, shiny skin that feels heavy for its size. It should be firm with a little spongy softness, but it shouldn't be too hard (overmature) or too soft (going bad). Avoid unusually small or large zucchini and instead stick to average-size squashes.

Storage: Remove any excess moisture with a paper towel and store in the crisper drawer of your refrigerator for up to five to seven days.

Preparation: The skin of squash has the highest concentration of nutrients, so leave it on. Slice up raw summer squash and dip into a tapenade or guacamole. For a warm dish, steam or sauté quickly for about three minutes. You can also spiralize it into pasta or add cubes to an omelet. As with other vegetables, avoid microwaving or boiling squash—it causes significant antioxidant loss.

Avoid overly large or small sized squashes.

Should feel firm with a bit of give.

CHAPTER 5

GRAINS

Many people love grain-based foods and eat them on a regular basis. The good news is that whole grains can be a wonderful addition to a healthy diet. But the bad news is that we're largely consuming refined grains, which do not support our health.

Here's why: Refined grains are high in calories, low in nutrients, and high glycemic, which all inevitably contribute to weight gain. Whole grains, on the other hand, are generally a good source of fiber, B vitamins, and minerals including iron, selenium, and magnesium. A 2007 USDA report found that 93 percent of Americans failed to consume the recommended three ounces (85 g) of whole grains daily. Instead, we consume more than five ounces (140 g) of refined grains daily—77 percent more than the USDA suggests.

This chapter shows you why it's important to choose the correct types and preparation methods if you include grains in your diet. In general, whole grains are preferable to refined grains, and gluten-free grains are preferable to those that contain gluten.

Regarding preparation, you'll want to learn more about the seldom used—but highly beneficial—techniques of sprouting and fermenting. And here's some more good news: No matter what your favorite refined-grain food is, you can rest assured there's probably a healthier, gluten-free, whole-grain version of it.

Grain Buzzwords

Multiple words are used to describe grains. Here's help deciphering what they mean.

WHOLE GRAIN

A whole grain is a cereal grain that contains the germ, endosperm, and bran layers and, therefore, the protein, fiber, and nutrients contained in them. Examples of whole grains include brown rice and steel cut oats. Be warned, though, that sometimes you'll see a product—bread, perhaps—with a label that says it's made with "whole grain." This doesn't necessarily mean the product is made *solely* with whole grain. So always double check the ingredients list to see if it also contains refined grains, such as white or enriched flour, which sometimes hide in "whole-grain" products. From a health standpoint, the addition of refined grains makes a product less desirable.

REFINED GRAINS

These are grains that have had their germ and bran layers removed, which also removes much of the protein, fiber, and nutrients normally found in them. Refined grains are typically white in color, like white flour, white bread, or white rice. The labels of refined-grain products won't actually use the phrase "refined grains," but you'll know they're refined if they contain white flour.

ENRICHED/FORTIFIED

This label identifies a highly processed refined-grain product that's had its natural nutrients stripped out during processing. They are then replaced with synthetic vitamins. In my opinion, enriched-grain products are inferior to whole, unprocessed grains that naturally contain nutrients.

GLUTEN

This is a protein found in wheat and certain other grains and grain products that many people find hard to digest. It has been associated with inflammation, damage to the intestinal lining, fatigue, and other health problems.

GLUTEN FREE

A gluten-free grain or product does not contain wheat or other gluten-containing grains. Gluten-free grains may be easier to digest for some people. In the whole foods or bulk section of the market, it can be hard to tell which grains contain gluten and which don't, so check the chart on page 122 to see which ones are gluten free.

In the packaged foods section, remember that just because a product is gluten free doesn't mean it's healthy. For instance, a gluten-free cookie is still a cookie.

SPROUTED

Sprouting is a method of soaking a grain in water for a period of time to make it easier to digest and increase the amount and bioavailability of the nutrients it contains. Sprouted grains are ideal for good health.

FERMENTED

Fermented grains have been fermented with yeast or bacteria, which gives them their signature sour flavor. Fermented grains are easier to digest for many people and also tend to be more nutritious because fermentation reduces phytic acid and makes the grains' natural minerals more available for absorption. Sourdough is a good example.

Benefits of Grains

Beyond tasting good, whole grains provide a variety of health benefits. Here are their best-known qualities:

REDUCE HEART DISEASE & STROKE RISK

According to the Whole Grains Council, regularly consuming whole grains—not refined grains—reduces the risk of heart disease by at least 25 percent and reduces the risk of stroke by at least 30 percent.

SUPPORT DIGESTIVE HEALTH & IMPROVE REGULARITY

Whole grains are a good source of fiber, which promotes regularity and lowers your risk of colorectal cancer.

REDUCED RISK OF TYPE 2 DIABETES

Regular consumption of whole grains may lower the risk of type 2 diabetes by 21 to 30 percent, according to the Whole Grains Council.

AID IN WEIGHT LOSS

Epidemiological studies consistently indicate that higher intakes of whole grains (but not refined grains) are associated with a lower body mass index (BMI)—a measure of weight based on height—and/or a reduced risk of obesity. Numerous observational studies have shown that consuming about three servings of whole grains a day is associated with less belly fat and less risk of weight gain compared to nonconsumption.

Concerns About Grains

Grains in their whole form are health supportive, but when they are highly processed and refined into convenience foods, such as bread and pasta, they raise a number of health concerns. Additionally, grains that contain gluten may also be problematic. Here is what you should know:

REFINED GRAINS

All grains begin as whole grains in nature. They're composed of three layers:

1. The germ, which contains B vitamins, some protein, minerals, and healthy fats

2. The bran, which contains important antioxidants, B vitamins, and fiber

3. The endosperm, which contains starchy carbohydrates, proteins, and small amounts of vitamins and minerals

Because whole grains contain all three layers, they're high in protein, fiber, vitamins, minerals, and antioxidants. These nutrient-rich complex carbs allow for the slow absorption of sugar into your bloodstream, providing long-lasting energy to keep you fueled for hours. Refined grains, though, are a different story, and they're the reason grains, or "carbs," get such a bad rap.

Refined grains have been processed to remove their bran and germ layers, leaving just the endosperm. This strips the grain of much of its fiber; about 25 percent of its protein; and at least 17 key nutrients. You can easily spot refined grains by their color—white, as in white bread, white rice, or white flour, which is used in many types of pasta and baked goods.

Aside from being less nutritious, refined grains are also higher glycemic, which means

❗ Expert Tip

Avoid high glycemic foods for weight loss. High glycemic foods spike blood sugar, while low glycemic foods keep it stable. A high glycemic diet, one that consists mostly of refined foods, such as bread, cereal, pasta, baked goods, and sugary foods, is associated with an increased risk of weight gain, while a low glycemic diet (or real-food diet, filled with whole foods) is associated with weight loss and maintenance.

they're more quickly digested into simple sugars and absorbed into your bloodstream, causing blood sugar levels to spike and then crash quickly. These rapid swings in blood sugar can be the culprit behind weight gain; they may also drain your energy and leave you feeling moody and tired. Avoid refined grains and stick to whole grains.

INSTANT GRAINS

Instant grains have been processed or precooked to minimize cooking time for the consumer. Grains processed or milled in this way, such as one-minute oatmeal, are still technically "whole grains" as they still contain their three layers. But, because they've been subjected to additional processing, they have more surface area, which allows them to cook faster. This also means your body will digest them more quickly, causing more of a blood sugar spike than unprocessed grains would. Instant grains also tend to be slightly lower in nutrients than their unprocessed counterparts.

Precooked whole grains, such as frozen brown rice, can be a good option. This simply cuts cooking time without changing the surface area of the grain.

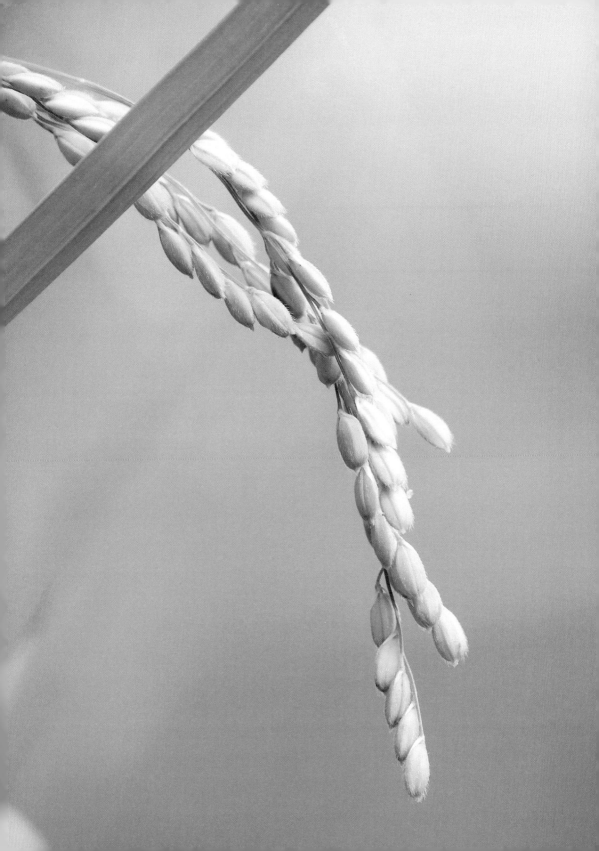

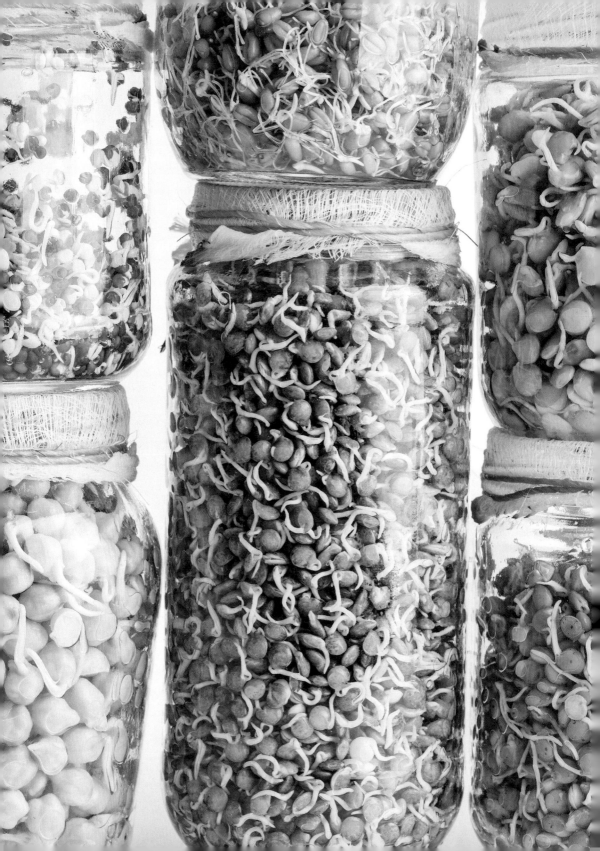

How to Sprout Grains: Step by Step

You can sprout any whole grain, but not those that are hulled, pearled, rolled, or otherwise processed. One-half cup of dry grains yields about two cups sprouted. (Weights vary among grains.)

Consume sprouted grains within a few days. If they get slimy or smelly, discard them. Sprouts can be subject to contamination. If the original grain or seed is contaminated, bacteria such as E. coli may grow, which could cause food-borne illnesses. Always purchase organic fresh products from a reputable source and cook sprouted grains before you consume them. The sprouting process should reduce the cooking time considerably and the amount of water required, but this varies from grain to grain.

Amaranth: one to three days
Barley: two days
Buckwheat: two to three days
Millet: twelve hours
Oats: two to three days
Quinoa: two to three days
Wild rice: three to five days

Follow these simple steps to sprout your own grains.

1. **Soak the grains.** In a large bowl, combine two cups (475 ml) warm water plus one tablespoon (15 ml) apple cider vinegar or fresh lemon juice. Add one-half cup (weights vary) grains, cover the bowl, and soak overnight or at least eight hours. Sprouted grains are highly perishable; soak only what you will use in the next few days.

2. **Drain and rinse.** Pour the grains into a colander and rinse well.

3. **Prepare a sprouting container.** Sprouts need space and air, so if sprouting a large batch, you'll need a few one-quart (946 ml) Mason jars. Use about one-half cup (weights vary) grains per one-quart (946 ml) jar. Cover the jar with a double layer of cheesecloth secured with a rubber band or the jar's metal ring lid. (Do not use the solid metal lid insert.)

4. **Sprout the grains.** In a bowl, turn the jar upside down and rest it at an angle so air can circulate and water can drain out. Keep it at room temperature, out of direct light.

5. **Rinse and drain twice a day.** Every twelve hours or so, pour water into the jar and swirl it to rinse the grains. Then dump out the water and let it sit again, inverted and at an angle.

6. **Wait and watch.** You'll know they've sprouted when you see little "tails" emerge. Use them now or let the tails grow to a quarter inch (6 mm). Refrigerate sprouted grains if not using right away.

- Amaranth
- Buckwheat
- Millet
- Oats*
- Quinoa
- Rice (all types)
- Sorghum
- Teff

*Oats are a gluten-free grain, but they're easily cross-contaminated during harvest and processing. Choose those with a certified gluten-free seal. These should be fine for most people, but if you have celiac disease, you should avoid them as they've been known to trigger a similar reaction to gluten—the exact cause of which is not known.

GLUTEN

Gluten is a type of protein found in certain grains, particularly wheat. It has been associated with a whole host of problems, including digestive issues, weight gain, skin disorders, low energy, autoimmune conditions, and brain fog. Plus, both test tube and human studies have demonstrated that gluten can trigger the immune system, spark inflammation, and increase intestinal permeability (also known as leaky gut). This can occur whether or not you've been diagnosed with celiac disease or a gluten sensitivity or allergy. Research on the negative effects of gluten is continuing, so, to be on the safe side, choose naturally gluten-free grains.

HARD TO DIGEST

If they are not chosen or prepared correctly, grains can be hard for some people to digest. To make grains gentler on the digestive system, choose gluten-free grains and ferment or sprout them before cooking.

Because grains are the seeds of cereal grasses, if you provide them with the ideal temperature and moisture and a sufficient amount of time, they'll begin to sprout into a plant. Historically, grains would have sprouted naturally when left out in the rain after harvesting, but these days, our modern processing methods have eliminated that possibility. That's unfortunate because, as it turns out, sprouted grains offer a number of benefits, so some manufacturers—and individuals—have started to sprout grains again.

GRAINS & THE PALEO DIET

With the growing popularity of the Paleo, or "caveman," style of eating, grains have fallen out of favor, and there's been a shift toward eliminating grains from the diet altogether. According to Paleo proponents, our ancestors didn't eat grains and they should be avoided due to their phytate (also known as phytic acid), lectin, and gluten content. Apart from the fact that anthropologists have found evidence that our ancestors did, indeed, ingest grains, the fact that grains contain these three antinutrients doesn't necessarily indicate they should be avoided completely.

Here's why. First, phytates are not inherently damaging, but they do bind with minerals and prevent their absorption. They shouldn't concern people whose diets are rich in minerals, especially when grains are prepared properly. Soaking them in water with lemon juice or vinegar before cooking greatly reduces the phytate content.

As for lectins, they're found in raw grains and legumes and, to a lesser extent, nuts, seeds, and even certain fruits and vegetables. If they were really such a threat, we'd also have to cut out carrots, zucchini, melon, grapes, cherries, raspberries, blackberries, garlic, and mushrooms (among others)—all of which contain lectins, but are given the thumbs up according to Paleo protocol.

The main concern with ingesting lectins, according to Paleo advocates, is that test tube and animal studies have demonstrated a link between lectins and damage to the gut lining, which could potentially lead to autoimmune diseases. But this is a weak argument for several reasons. First, because a food contains thousands of phytochemicals, a test tube study investigating the effects of a single component isn't necessarily a good gauge of how it will affect the human body when ingested. Second, the animal study often cited by Paleo proponents that links lectins to gut damage involved the consumption of excessive amounts of raw legumes. It's unlikely that any human would ingest such a large quantity— and even if they did, the legumes would almost certainly have been cooked, which reduces lectin content. (Soaking, sprouting, or fermenting grains reduces lectin content even further.) Third, several lectins have been found to possess anticancer properties in test tube and human studies, so they may not be so bad after all. It's also possible that the many other nutrients in grains may offset any potentially negative effects of lectins.

In short, when properly prepared gluten-free grains comprise a small part of a healthy person's real-food diet, they may not be problematic. However, if you suffer from leaky gut or an autoimmune condition, it can't hurt to experiment with removing grains completely from your diet to see whether it makes a difference for you.

ARSENIC IN RICE

In 2012, *Consumer Reports* released its analysis of arsenic in rice products. Inorganic arsenic—a carcinogen—and organic arsenic, which is less toxic but still of concern, was found in all the rice products tested, including white rice, brown rice, and foods made from them, such as cereal, baby food, and snack foods. The presence of arsenic in children's food is most troubling, as it can pose risks to brain development.

However, rice is not the only food found to contain arsenic. It's been identified in fruit, vegetables, juice, meat, and even water. The Environmental Protection Agency (EPA) assumes there is no safe level of exposure to inorganic arsenic, and no federal limit exists. The standard for drinking water is ten parts per billion (ppb), although the EPA originally proposed five ppb as a maximum.

In some cases, brown rice—which is nutritionally superior to white rice thanks to its additional fiber, vitamins, and minerals—had as much as 50 to 100 percent more inorganic arsenic in a single serving than the recommended 5 ppb, which could cause problems for people who regularly consume these products. Some of the worst offenders were health foods made from brown rice, such as pasta, syrup, and rice cakes.

White rice, on the other hand, contained arsenic, but less than 5 ppb per serving—presumably because some of the arsenic was removed along with the rice's outer layers during processing. Rice grown in other countries, including India and Thailand, had much lower levels than U.S.-grown rice, according to the analysis. Rice from Arkansas, Louisiana, Missouri, and Texas tended to have the highest arsenic concentrations, while rice grown in California had lower concentrations.

Where Does the Arsenic Originate?

A limited amount may occur naturally in the soil, but according to *Consumer Reports*,

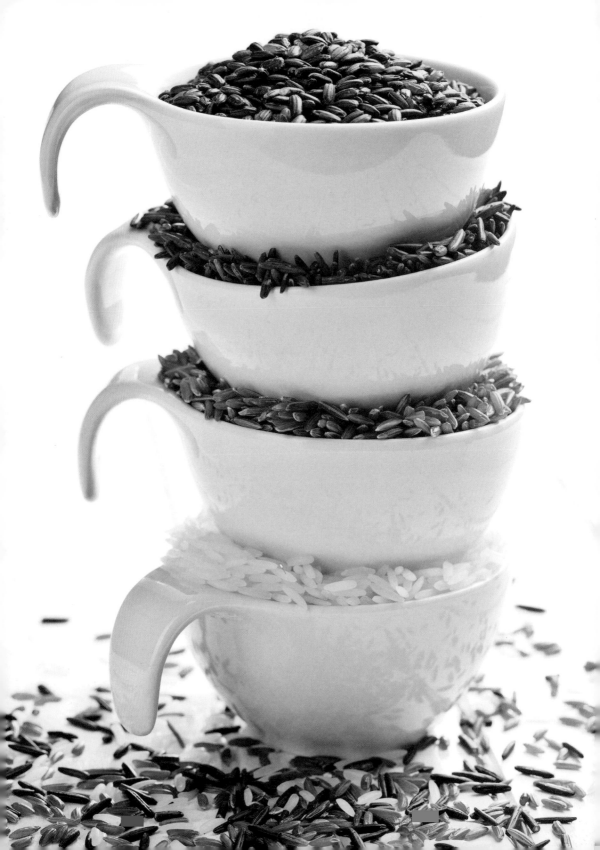

American agricultural practices are mostly to blame. Since 1910, 1.6 million tons (1.45 million metric tons) of arsenic have been used for agricultural and industrial purposes, making the United States the world's leading user of arsenic. Its use was banned in the 1980s, but residue from decades of use remains in the soil. Up until 2015, arsenic was permitted for use in livestock feed (it promotes growth), so fertilizer made from poultry waste could contaminate crops with inorganic arsenic. This situation demonstrates why it's smart to choose organic foods whenever you can to promote more sustainable farming practices. The decisions we make now don't only affect

◎ Myth Alert!

Myth: All carbs are bad.

Fact: Not all carbs are bad because not all carbs are created equal.

It's important to distinguish between the nutrient called "carbohydrates" from the term "carbohydrates," which is sometimes used interchangeably with "grains." As nutrients, carbs are an important part of a healthy diet. They are the primary energy source for our brains and critical to the functioning of the central nervous system, kidneys, heart, and muscles. Some of the healthiest foods—namely, fruits and vegetables—contain carbs.

When referring to grains as carbs, choose unrefined over refined carbs. Refined carbs, such as white bread and white flour, are best avoided. They're associated with negative health outcomes, including weight gain and diabetes. Unrefined carbs, or whole grains, are associated with such health benefits as lower risks for diabetes, weight gain, and cardiovascular disease. You don't have to—and shouldn't!—avoid all carbs. *Avoid only those carbs that come from refined grains.*

❶ Expert Tip

How to Choose Grains

- Choose whole, not refined, grains—ideally sprouted or fermented.
- Choose naturally gluten-free grains, such as amaranth, buckwheat, millet, oats, quinoa, rice (all types), sorghum, and teff.
- Avoid grains with gluten, such as wheat, barley, bulgur, durum, farro, kamut, rye, semolina, spelt, and triticale.

our lives, but also the well-being of generations to come.

Still, when consumed in moderation—and from, less contaminated sources—a little rice here and there probably doesn't present much cause for concern. To avoid or limit your exposure, choose white rice grown in California, India, and Thailand and limit your overall consumption of rice products.

Gluten-Free Grains

There are numerous naturally gluten-free grains that are also delicious! Some may be unfamiliar to you, but all are generally inexpensive and easy to prepare—be on the lookout for new recipes to try them in.

AMARANTH

An ancient grain that was a staple of Aztec culture, amaranth is a complete protein, loaded with a variety of minerals, including calcium and iron. It's a good source of fiber, which aids digestion and may help lower cholesterol and support overall heart health. Amaranth can be made into a side dish or breakfast porridge.

BLACK RICE

Dubbed "forbidden rice" because it was reserved for royalty in ancient Asia, this rice gets its inky black color from anthocyanins, potent antioxidants being studied for their anticancer potential. Black rice contains more protein and fiber than any other type of rice, making it the most filling and satisfying variety.

BROWN RICE

This health-food-restaurant staple is an excellent source of manganese and a good source of selenium, phosphorus, copper, magnesium, and niacin. Whole grains, such as brown rice, aid in maintaining a healthy body weight and lowering cholesterol. There are numerous varieties, including short grain (which is fuller and chewier), long grain, and jasmine brown rice. Add a few sliced mushrooms to a pot of cooking brown rice for an instant flavor boost. Choose varieties grown in India, Thailand, or California to limit your arsenic exposure, as discussed previously (see page 123).

BUCKWHEAT

Although used like a grain, buckwheat is actually a seed. It contains a specific antioxidant—rutin—that studies show improves circulation and supports cardiovascular health. You can turn the seed into a breakfast porridge or use buckwheat flour to make pancakes and breads. It's used in many traditional dishes across the world, including Japanese soba noodles, French crêpes, and Russian kasha.

MILLET

Often overlooked in Western culture, millet is a staple in many other parts of the world. It is quick cooking and extremely versatile. It can be made into a creamy polenta, a fluffy whole grain, a delicious breakfast porridge, nutritious breads, and even healthy desserts. It has a

◎ **Myth Alert!**

Myth: White rice is bad and should never be eaten because it's a refined carb.

Fact: It's okay to eat white rice if you pair it with beans or other legumes.

While it's true that white rice is refined, and that refined grains aren't healthy in general, white rice is an exception when paired with the right foods. Eating white rice by itself is a recipe for an unhealthy blood sugar spike. However, when you pair it with protein- and fiber-rich beans or lentils, as in traditional Indian and Latin American dishes, you lower the overall glycemic index of the meal, preventing the large blood sugar spike associated with eating white rice on its own. While it's not something you'll want to eat every day—there are many more nutritious options!—if you pair it with lentils or beans, white rice is an exception to the "no refined grains" rule.

nutty, slightly corn-like flavor and is loaded with minerals, including copper, phosphorus, manganese, and magnesium. Toast it briefly in a hot, dry pan before cooking to get the best flavor.

OATS

A satisfying, fiber-rich breakfast choice, oats support healthy digestion and keep you feeling full for hours. Some studies suggest that their beta-glucan content also supports a strong immune system. For the highest nutrition and satiety, always choose steel-cut or Irish-style oats (which take thirty minutes to prepare) or rolled oats (which take five minutes to prepare) and, ideally, choose a brand certified gluten-free to avoid cross-contamination. Instant oatmeal is typically lower in fiber, protein, and nutrients and is also higher glycemic, so it's best avoided.

QUINOA

Quinoa, another seed often mistaken for a grain, is a complete plant protein that takes just ten to fifteen minutes to prepare. It's light, fluffy, and has a neutral flavor, so it's easy to dress it up any way you want. It contains a variety of minerals and antioxidants, and although you'll typically find the white variety in most stores, it's also available in red, purple, and black. Prepare it as a side dish or breakfast bowl; add it to salads for a plant-based protein; or use it in baked goods.

RED RICE

Red rice contains ten times more antioxidants than brown rice and slightly more fiber, too. The red color comes from anthocyanins—potent antioxidants. Use it in place of white or brown rice.

SORGHUM

An ancient African grain, sorghum can be popped like popcorn, cooked into porridge, or ground into flour for use in baked goods. Studies show that sorghum may help manage cholesterol and protect against diabetes and insulin resistance. Darker sorghum contains more antioxidants than lighter varieties, and some preliminary test tube studies suggest it may inhibit tumor growth.

TEFF

This teeny-tiny grain contains more iron and calcium than any other. Teff has a sweet, molasses-like flavor and can be used in porridges, breads, baked goods, or to make "polenta." It's the principal grain used in spongy Ethiopian *injera* bread.

WHITE RICE

White rice is brown rice minus its outer layers, making it much easier to digest—and much less nutritious. Although it is, in fact, a refined carb, check out the Myth Alert! on page 126 to learn how it can be an exception to the "no refined grains" rule.

❗ **Expert Tip**

Suggested Serving Size Guidelines for Grains	
Serving size	One-half cup (about 100 g) cooked
Servings per day	Up to three
Frequency per week	Daily, or as you wish. Although grains contain nutrients, those nutrients can be found in other foods—namely, vegetables. So, as they require extra preparation for sprouting and fermenting, fill your plate with more vegetables than grains on some—even most—days.

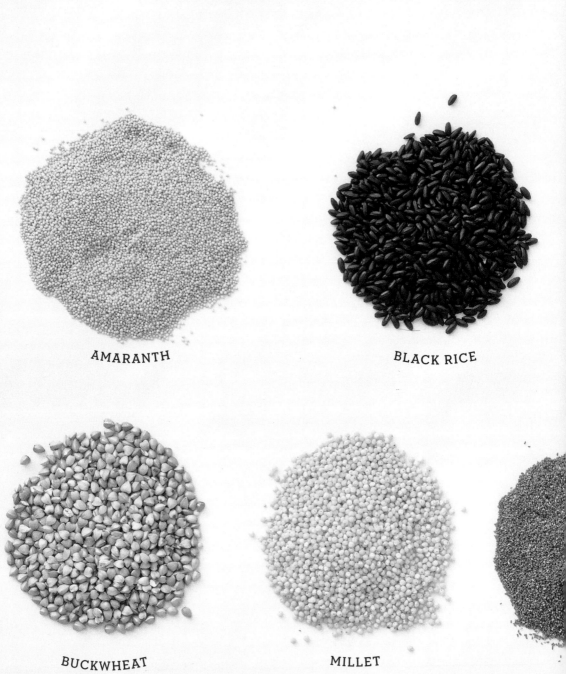

AMARANTH

BLACK RICE

BUCKWHEAT

MILLET

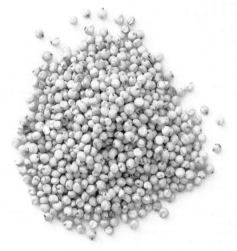

SORGHUM

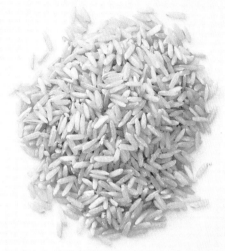

BROWN RICE

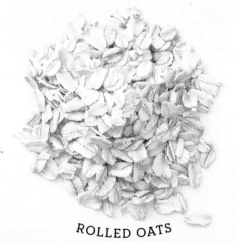

TEFF

ROLLED OATS

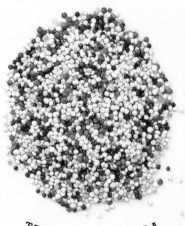

TRI-COLOR QUINOA

CHAPTER 6

LEGUMES, BEANS & SOY

Legumes, including beans, peas, and lentils, have always been grouped with "protein" in the USDA's Food Pyramid and MyPlate. But in my opinion, they deserve their own food group because they're very different from meat and much more nutritious. (In fact, in Brazil they're considered a separate food group to be eaten each day.)

Legumes come in a wide variety of colors, shapes, and sizes and can be purchased dry or precooked in cans or jars or even frozen. Homemade beans are often the tastiest—yet prepackaged varieties do offer timesaving convenience. Still, because of concern over toxins in can linings (as you'll learn in chapter 12), consider limiting your intake of canned legumes and choose other forms of packaged varieties instead. (Although peanuts are also part of the legume family, they're discussed in chapter 7, which focuses on nuts and seeds, because they're often thought of and treated like nuts.)

Likely you're aware of beans' better-known attribute—thanks to a certain charming childhood rhyme. (Beans, beans, they're good for your heart. The more you eat, the more you—well, you know how it goes!) But these miniature nutritional powerhouses haven't received the (positive) spotlight they deserve—until now, that is. And the good news is when you eat them regularly, you'll be better able to digest them, so they won't act like the "musical fruit" they're thought to be.

Legumes, Beans & Soy Buzzwords

When purchasing legumes, beans, or soy, following are the terms you should be familiar with:

LEGUME

Beans, peas, and lentils are all part of the legume family.

DRIED

Typically found in the bulk sections of groceries, dried beans are uncooked beans. Canned beans, in contrast, are cooked and ready to use. Dried beans should be soaked overnight and then cooked—ideally in a pressure cooker (see page 134).

SPROUTED

You can now find sprouted and dried beans and lentils for sale in health food stores. Sprouted legumes tend to be easier to digest and more nutritious, too. They still need to be cooked, though they may require less water or cooking time than unsprouted legumes. Follow package directions.

BPA-FREE CANS

BPA-free cans were once considered a healthier alternative to cans containing BPA, a chemical linked to hormone disruption and serious health problems, including heart disease and cancer. However, it turns out that BPC and BPS, the alternative chemicals used in BPA-free cans, are just as toxic as BPA—perhaps even more so—and best avoided. (See chapter 12 for a more in-depth discussion.)

NON-GMO

When purchasing any type of soy, you may see it marked "non-GMO." This indicates it was not genetically modified (see chapter 12, for a more in-depth discussion of GMOs). Organic soy is automatically non-GMO (although, non-GMO soy is not automatically organic).

Benefits of Legumes & Beans

Beans and legumes can be an incredibly nutritious addition to your diet. Here are some of their top benefits:

WEIGHT LOSS

Legumes are extremely high in fiber and protein, yet relatively low in calories, making them excellent foods for weight loss. On average, one cup (about 180 g) of beans—such as black beans—contains about fifteen grams of protein, fifteen grams of fiber, and slightly more than two hundred calories.

CARDIOVASCULAR HEALTH

A diet high in legumes can help prevent cardiovascular disease and lower cholesterol. Canadian researchers saw a 5 percent reduction in bad LDL cholesterol in as little as six weeks in mostly middle-aged men and women who ate one serving (¾ cup, or about 135 g) of beans per day. A study in the *Archives of Internal Medicine* that followed almost ten-thousand adults over nineteen years found those who ate the most fiber—twenty-one grams per day—had 12 percent less coronary heart disease and 11 percent less cardiovascular disease compared to those who ate the least (5 g daily).

Research has also shown that swapping meat for legumes likely lowers the risk of cardiovascular disease. One prospective cohort study that followed participants for nineteen years found those who ate legumes at least four times a week had a 21 percent lower risk of coronary heart disease than those who ate them less than once a week.

BALANCE BLOOD SUGAR

In a small study published in the *Journal of the American Medical Association*, researchers found that, compared with a diet rich in whole grains, a daily dose of legumes led to improved glycemic control. So, downing a cup of beans or lentils (about 180 to 200 g) every day may help people with type 2 diabetes control their blood sugar and may help others lose weight or maintain a healthy weight.

RICH IN MINERALS

Legumes are an excellent source of phytonutrients and many minerals, including iron, which is needed for energy; folate, crucial to brain and nervous system health; and molybdenum, which promotes antioxidant protection and detoxification.

How to Make a Complete Plant-Based Protein

If your diet is solely plant-based, make sure you consume complete proteins every day. To make a complete plant-based protein, you need to consume at least one serving of any of these food combinations—not necessarily at the same meal, just within the same twenty-four-hour period.

- Legume + Grain
- Legume + Nuts
- Legume + Seeds

CANCER PROTECTION

Fiber is believed to play a role in reducing the risk of certain types of cancer, so it should come as no surprise that fiber-rich legumes have been linked to cancer prevention. Studies have shown that higher legume intake is associated with a lower risk of colorectal, stomach, and kidney cancers.

PLANT-BASED PROTEIN

Think you have to eat meat to get protein? Think again. Most plant-based foods, including vegetables and fruits, have at least some protein. However, legumes are the richest sources, delivering an average of about fifteen grams per cup (about 180 g).

Protein plays a crucial role in our bodies and is responsible for cell function and health. Proteins are made up of a combination of up to twenty amino acids. Nine of the twenty are *essential*—meaning we need to consume them, through food, every day.

Foods that contain all nine essential amino acids are called *complete proteins*. Examples include black beans, cashews, chia seeds, chickpeas, hemp seeds, kidney beans, pistachios, pumpkin seeds, quinoa, and soy. The remaining eleven amino acids can either be consumed in other foods or are produced by our bodies. While all animal products are complete proteins, only some plant-based foods are. This is probably part of the reason many people (wrongly) assume you can't get sufficient protein from plant-based foods alone. That's not true. Because they contain complementary amino acids, incomplete proteins such as beans can be paired with other incomplete proteins—nuts, seeds, or grains—to form complete proteins.

Concerns About Legumes & Beans

Although beans have many health benefits, it's important that they are properly prepared to mitigate health concerns, such as gas, bloating, and anti-nutrients. For those who follow a 100 percent plant-based diet and rely on beans and legumes for protein, combine them with other foods to create a complete protein.

LEGUMES, ANTINUTRIENTS & THE PALEO DIET

As with grains, people who follow the Paleo diet avoid all legumes on the grounds they contain toxic antinutrients called lectins and phytic acid. Legumes do, in fact, contain lectins and phytic acid, but it's unlikely they're a cause for concern. Let me explain.

First, let's look at lectins. Studies have, indeed, shown they can impair growth, damage the lining of the small intestine, destroy skeletal muscle, and interfere with the function of the pancreas. But these studies were conducted with animals consuming massive amounts of raw legumes. Humans wouldn't eat nearly as much—and we definitely wouldn't eat them raw. Cooking legumes for just fifteen minutes almost completely inactivates the lectins they contain, and beans are typically soaked and cooked for hours.

As for phytic acid, Paleo proponents argue we cannot digest it and that it binds to minerals and prevents us from absorbing them. (It doesn't leach minerals present in our bodies; it just blocks absorption of the minerals in the foods we consume.) This is true, but it isn't the whole picture.

Human cells may not be able to break down phytic acid, but our gut bacteria can. Plus, additional research shows that phytic acid acts as an antioxidant, prevents the accumulation of heavy metals in the body, and plays a role in cellular communication—so it may not be such a "bad" thing. What's more, many vegetables, including spinach and Swiss chard—as well as dark chocolate—contain two and three times the amount of phytic acid of legumes—but these foods are allowed on the Paleo diet, which doesn't make sense.

Last, the premise of eating Paleo is that we should eat like our ancestors did—and Paleo followers claim our Paleolithic ancestors did not consume legumes. But anthropologists have, in fact, found legumes in the digestive tracts of Paleolithic individuals. Now, this doesn't mean the entire Paleo diet is wrong: In fact, it's one of the healthier ways of eating. It simply means this particular component needs to be re-evaluated.

So, *must* you eat legumes? No. But if you don't, you will miss some amazing benefits.

BLOATING & GAS

If the mere thought of beans makes you gassy, it could be a sign your digestive flora simply isn't used to digesting legumes. It may take you a couple weeks to adjust, but there are a few simple ways to help beat bean bloat.

- Always soak beans. Then, ideally, use a pressure cooker to cook them. Not only does this reduce cooking time to minutes instead of hours, but it makes them especially easy to digest.

- While cooking beans, add a piece of kombu seaweed to the water. It absorbs some of the compounds that cause gas. Discard it after cooking.

- Take a multi-strain probiotic daily for at least thirty days to reseed your gut with good bacteria that may help you digest beans naturally and without discomfort.

- Start slowly. If you're not used to eating beans, start with ¼ cup (about 45 g), work up to ½ cup (about 90 g), ¾ cup (about 135 g), and so on over the course of a few weeks.

- Prepare the beans with carminative spices, such as cumin, coriander, anise seeds, or fennel. These spices are used in many traditional recipes and preparations to help combat flatulence.

INCOMPLETE PROTEIN

Though certain plant-based proteins are complete proteins—containing all essential amino acids we need daily—such as quinoa and soy, most, such as beans and lentils, are incomplete proteins that need to be paired with a grain, nut, or seed to deliver all the essential amino acids. If you eat a primarily plant-based diet, it's a good idea to get into the habit of eating beans or lentils with rice to ensure you get a complete protein.

Cooking Dried Beans

Cooking dried beans takes a little forethought—they require overnight soaking and hours of boiling, but minimal effort. Beans freeze well, however, so consider cooking a large batch and freezing the leftovers.

Using a pressure cooker is ideal for cooking beans. Not only does it cut cooking time drastically (though you still have to soak the beans) and make them easier to digest, it allows them to retain more antioxidants than when boiled.

The pressure cooking times below are approximate and based on the use of a high pressure setting and natural release method with presoaked beans. Actual times may vary depending on the pressure cooker.

1. **Sort the beans.** Pick through them and discard any pebbles, foreign particles, or discolored or shriveled beans.

2. **Rinse and soak the beans.** Drain and add them to a large pot and cover with fresh water by at least 2 inches (5 cm). One cup (about 194 g) dried beans yields about three cups (516 g) cooked. See the chart below for recommended times. Add spices, garlic, or onion at this point. Don't add salt until the beans are done cooking.

3. **Rinse and cook the beans.** Drain the beans, return to the pot, and refill the pot with fresh water. Bring to a boil, reduce the heat to low, and cover the pot. Cooking times may vary. Older beans can take longer to cook than fresher ones. Beans are done when they're tender yet firm.

Bean Type	Soaking Time	Stove-Top Cooking Time	Pressure Cooking Time (on High)
Aduki	8 hours*	45 minutes to 1 hour	4 minutes
Black, turtle	8 hours*	45 minutes to 1 hour	3 to 6 minutes
Cannellini (white kidney beans)	8 hours*	1½ hours	6 to 8 minutes
Chickpeas (garbanzo beans)	6 to 8 hours*	1½ to 2 hours	10 to 12 minutes
Green lentils	None	45 minutes to 1 hour	8 to 10 minutes
Green split peas	None	35 to 45 minutes	6 to 10 minutes
Kidney	6 to 8 hours*	1½ to 2 hours	5 to 8 minutes
Navy	6 to 8 hours*	1 to 1½ hours	3 to 4 minutes
Great Northern	6 to 8 hours*	45 minutes to 1 hour	4 to 8 minutes
Pinto	6 to 8 hours*	1 to 1½ hours	1 to 3 minutes
Red lentils	None	10 to 15 minutes	4 to 6 minutes
Small red	6 to 8 hours*	1 to 1½ hours	15 to 20 minutes

*or overnight

Types of Beans

Beans are known for their fiber and protein content, but you may be surprised to learn they're also a top source of antioxidants, which slow or prevent cell damage and, therefore, also slow aging and disease. Each type of bean has its own unique flavor and benefits.

CHICKPEAS

Chickpeas are particularly beneficial for digestive health because they consist of up to 75 percent insoluble fiber. They have a nutty taste and a buttery texture. Toss them onto salads, turn them into hummus, or simmer in Indian-style sauces.

BLACK BEANS

Inky-colored black beans offer a variety of antioxidants, including anthocyanins, potent antioxidants that exhibit anticancer properties. Cook with garlic and spices to serve as a side; purée into a dip; or turn into veggie burgers.

KIDNEY BEANS

Kidney beans are loaded with trace minerals and antioxidants. In fact, they're one of the top sources of antioxidants—on par with blueberries! They're great in simmered dishes, such as chili, where they absorb the flavors of the broth, and they make a great meat substitute when seasoned with spices and ground in a food processor.

❗ Expert Tip

Several studies suggest that swapping just a few servings of meat each week for plant-based proteins, such as beans, peas, or lentils, is enough to lower your risk for cardiovascular disease and type 2 diabetes.

❸ Money-Saving Tip

Canned beans may be more convenient, but they are significantly more expensive and slightly less healthy than dried ones (due to the toxic chemicals in the can's lining). When you purchase dried beans, you save money and avoid toxic chemicals—and they taste better, too!

PINTO BEANS

Pinto beans look like tiny paint-splattered canvases when dried, but turn a beautiful shade of pink when cooked. They are one of the top sources of antioxidants among beans and happen to be very versatile. Use them in chili, soups, or blended with spices into a creamy spread.

NAVY BEANS

The navy bean's moniker is a testament to its superior nutrient profile. It got its name after serving as a main source of nutrition for the U.S. Navy in the late-nineteenth century. Small white navy beans are perfect for making baked beans and are delicious when sautéed with garlic and olive oil. They can also be puréed into a spread or a soup.

CANNELLINI BEANS

Creamy white cannellini beans are a staple of Italian cuisine and make an excellent side dish when simply sautéed with garlic and olive oil. Try sautéing them with escarole and garlic—an Italian classic. Because they have such a creamy texture, they are a great (and sneaky!) replacement for dairy in soups.

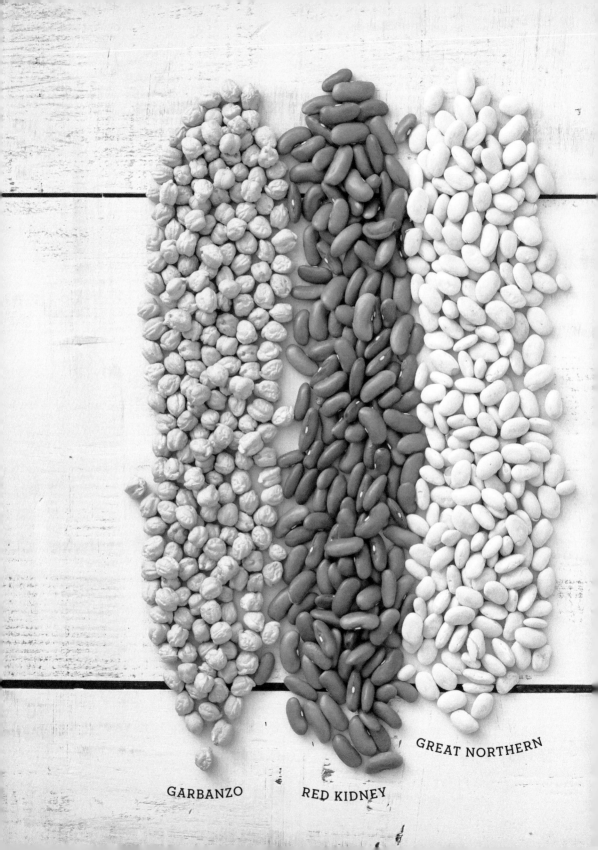

GARBANZO

RED KIDNEY

GREAT NORTHERN

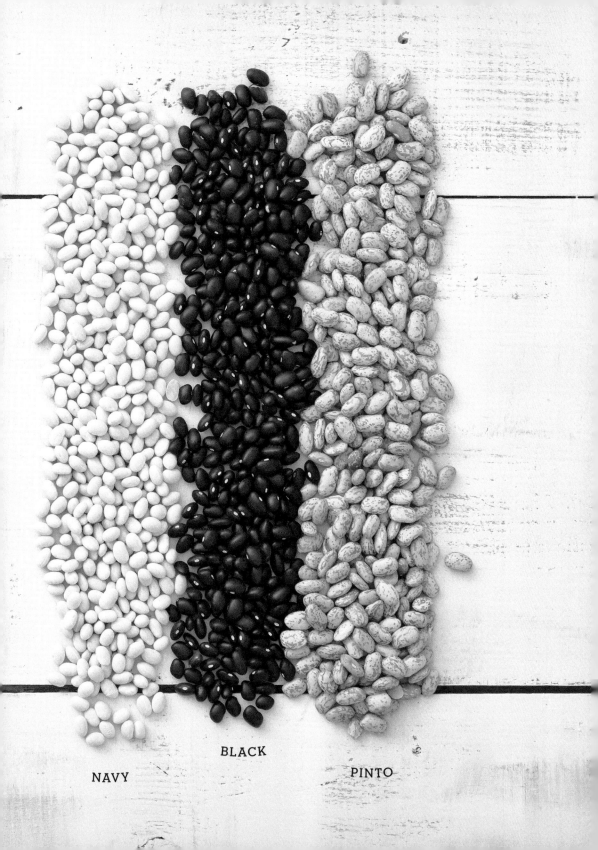

NAVY

BLACK

PINTO

GREAT NORTHERN BEANS

Great Northern beans are large white beans with a nutty flavor and creamy texture, which make them perfect in salads or soups or sautéed with garlic and veggies.

FAVA BEANS

Fava beans have a meaty, starchy texture that works well on its own or in soups, salads, or sides. In Egypt, they're cooked and then puréed with oil and spices for a savory breakfast called *ful medames*. In the spring, you can often find them fresh in their pods at farmers' markets.

Types of Lentils & Peas

Compared to other legumes, lentils are quick and easy to prepare. They're typically ready to eat in just twenty to forty minutes, from start to finish. There are many different types of lentils, but included here are some of the most common.

BLACK BELUGA LENTILS

The rich, earthy flavor and soft texture of these lentils make them perfect in salads and soups or with pasta, rice, or sautéed vegetables. Cook for twenty minutes if using firm in salads or up to thirty-five minutes for a more tender consistency.

BROWN LENTILS

Brown lentils are the most common type of lentil. With their mild, earthy flavor, they can be cooked and flavored many different ways. They hold their shape well and are ready in twenty to thirty minutes.

GREEN LENTILS/FRENCH LENTILS (DU PUY)

Although there are different types of green lentils, all of them have a slightly peppery flavor and hold their shape well, making them perfect for salads or side dishes. Of all the lentils, they take the longest to cook at about thirty to forty-five minutes.

RED LENTILS

Red lentils break down quickly during cooking and turn into a creamy golden-colored mush, so they're best used in soups or Indian-style dal dishes.

YELLOW LENTILS

Yellow lentils have a mild, nutty flavor. Like red lentils, they break down quickly and get soupy during cooking, so they're best suited to Indian-style dal dishes.

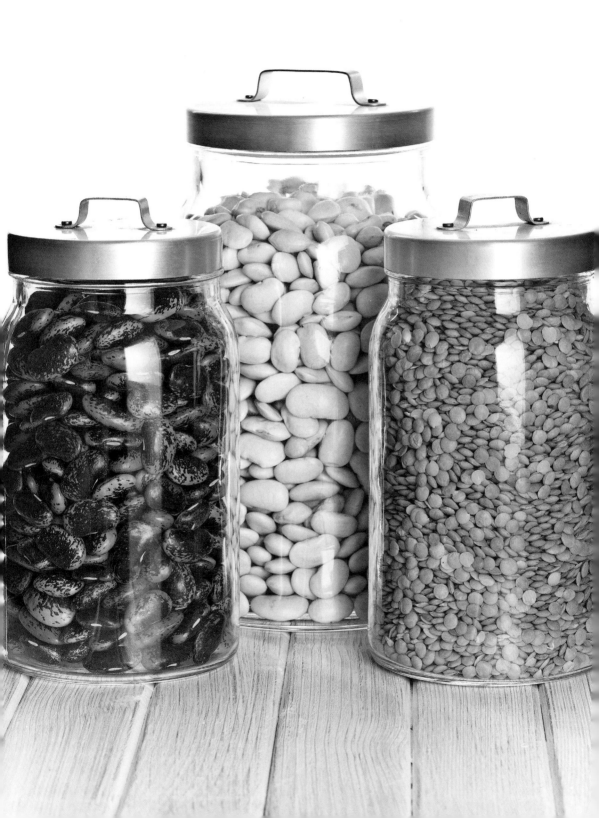

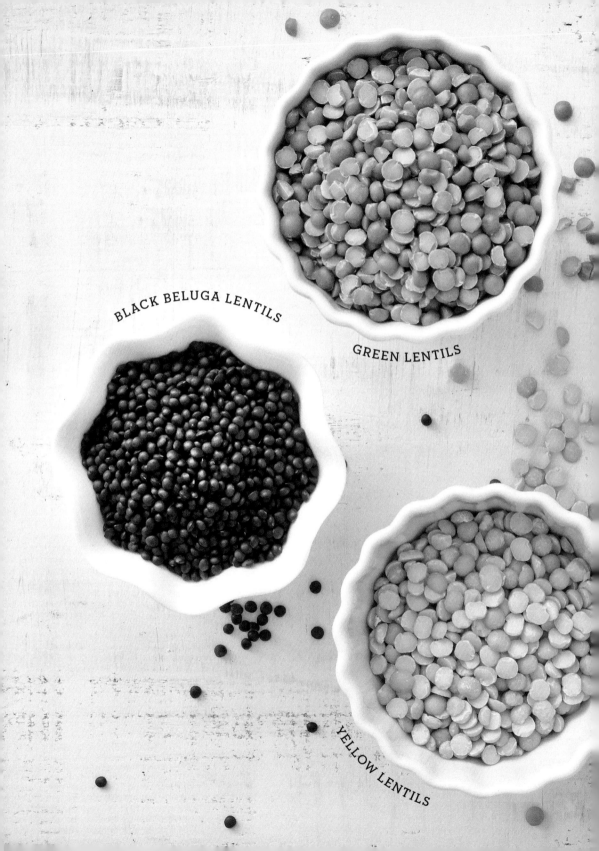

BLACK BELUGA LENTILS

GREEN LENTILS

YELLOW LENTILS

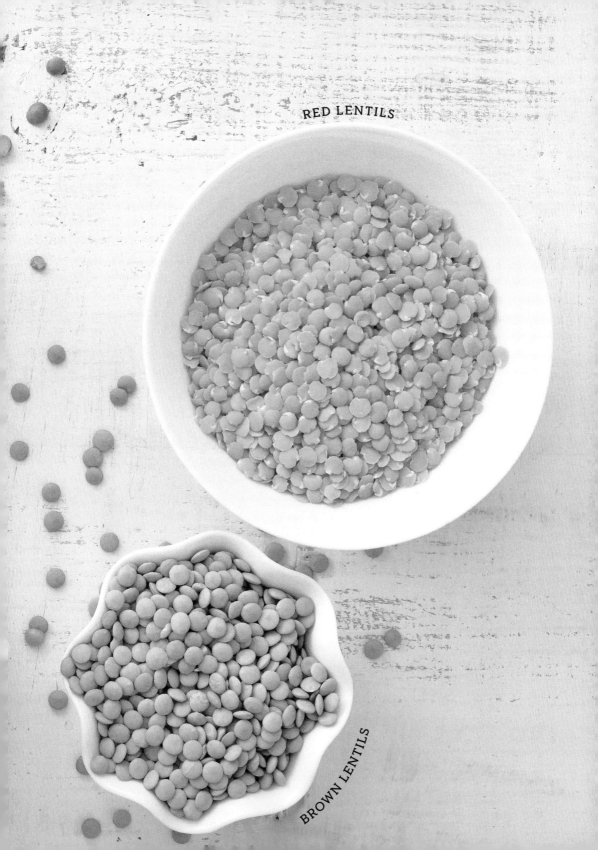

RED LENTILS

BROWN LENTILS

SPLIT PEAS

Split peas are a source of high-quality complete protein, which is especially important if you're following a plant-based diet. In addition to their high protein and fiber content, they contain a variety of minerals. Split peas are versatile when it comes to cooking. They'll retain their shape if cooked for a shorter period of time or will turn mushy when cooked longer, as they are in a typical Indian dal or split pea soup.

Soy

There's a lot of confusion about soy. Does it prevent cancer—or promote it? Much of the controversy stems from the fact it contains phytoestrogens (plant estrogens that mimic the female hormone in humans), which are incorrectly believed to promote estrogen-related cancers, such as breast cancer and endometrial cancer. However, not all soy is created equal, so there's no need to fear it— as long as you choose the right variety.

Benefits of Soy

Yes, soy has benefits! Note that any benefits mentioned are attributed to *unprocessed* or *fermented* soy—not to the highly processed soy typically found in packaged foods and protein shakes, which is the type of soy that gives the bean a bad rap.

SOY AND BREAST CANCER PREVENTION

In numerous human epidemiological studies that follow women over many years, results have consistently shown that soy has either no effect or a protective affect against breast cancer. This is true even for breast cancer survivors. A study published in the *Journal of The American Medical Association* that followed more than five thousand breast cancer survivors over five years found that "soy food consumption was significantly associated with decreased risk of death and recurrence."

COMPLETE PLANT-BASED PROTEIN

Unlike many types of beans and lentils, which are typically incomplete proteins, soy contains all the essential amino acids, making it a complete protein. For those following a 100 percent plant-based diet, including fermented soy in the diet can be an easy way to help you reach your daily protein needs.

SUPPORTS HEART HEALTH

Replacing commonly consumed animal protein products with soy foods aids in lowering LDL cholesterol by about 4 to 10 percent. In theory, over time, this may decrease the risk of coronary heart disease.

Concerns About Soy

The two most common misconceptions about soy have to do with men's health and thyroid health. Here's what you need to know:

SOY & MEN'S HEALTH

Soy is safe for consumption by men, and it will not alter their testosterone levels. In contrast to the results of some animal studies (which have given soy this bad reputation), human studies show that soy consumption will not feminize men. A meta-analysis of nine clinical studies published in the journal *Fertility and Sterility* found no evidence that soy had an effect on circulating estrogen levels or on sperm in men, and it was not found to be a cause of erectile dysfunction.

SOY & THYROID HEALTH

Clinical studies show that soy does not cause hypothyroidism. However, soy isoflavones may deplete some of the iodine the body would normally use to make thyroid hormones. Thus, people who eat soy must also consume adequate iodine, which can be found in sea vegetables, seafood, eggs, and iodized salt.

Types of Soy

According to the Physician's Committee for Responsible Medicine:

"Soy products are typically high in protein. Some manufacturers have exploited this fact, packing isolated soy protein into shakes and turning it into meat substitutes. However, it may be prudent to avoid highly concentrated proteins from any source, including soy. It has long been known that cow's milk increases the amount of insulin-like growth factor in the bloodstream, and this compound is linked to a cancer risk. Some evidence suggests that highly concentrated soy proteins (indicated as soy protein isolate on food labels) can do the same. Simple soy products, such as tempeh, edamame, or miso, are probably the best choices."

CHOOSE FERMENTED SOY

Fermented soy—tempeh, miso, natto, and soy sauce—has been a staple of Asian diets for thousands of years and is believed to be the healthiest way to consume soy. Like some other plant foods, soy naturally contains antinutrients, compounds that interfere with the absorption of minerals. However, when soy is fermented, these antinutrients are reduced, and the soy also becomes easier to digest, due to gas-causing compounds being reduced. Fermented soy is a great way to reap soy's health benefits. Choose only organic soy products to avoid GMOs.

CONSUME EDAMAME SPARINGLY

Edamame is unprocessed soy that may be hard to digest and contains antinutrients that block the absorption of minerals and nutrients. Although served regularly at Japanese restaurants, it's not a traditional food. Consume it sparingly or avoid it altogether.

AVOID PROCESSED SOY

Processed soy is refined so you're left with the protein and phytoestrogens—minus the antioxidants, vitamins, and other nutrients found in soy's whole, fermented form. It's found in many processed and packaged foods and is considered to be the least healthy form of soy. Examples include protein bars, protein shakes, soy cheese, soy ice cream, soy milk, soy protein isolate, soy yogurt, textured vegetable protein, and tofu. Consume this sparingly or avoid it completely.

❗ Expert Tip

Suggested Serving Size Guidelines for Legumes, Beans & Soy	
Serving size	One cup cooked lentils (198 g), beans (180 g), or peas, split (196 g); three ounces (85 g) tempeh
Servings per day	One to two
Frequency per week	Every day!

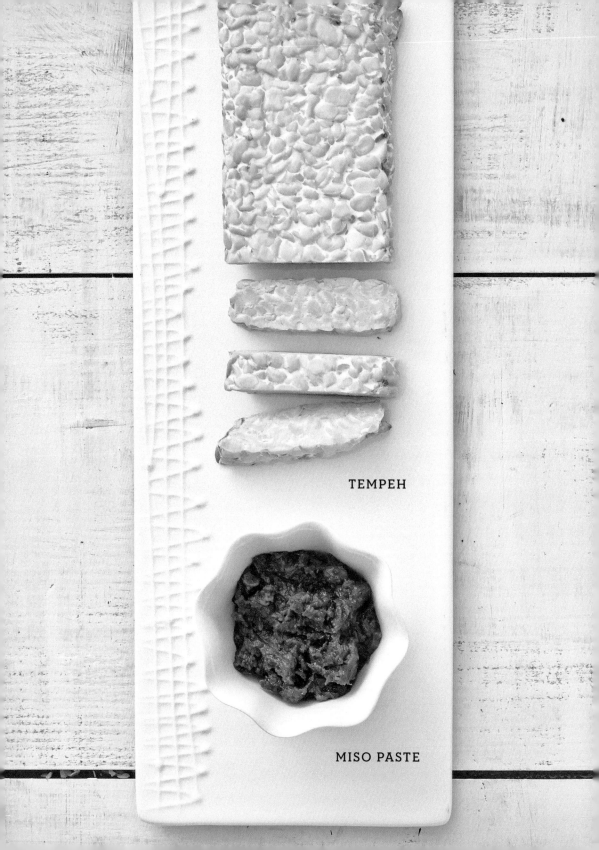

TEMPEH

MISO PASTE

EDAMAME

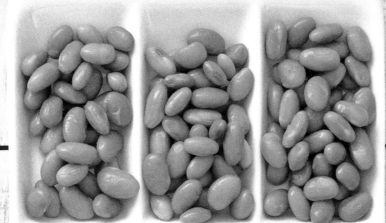

TOFU

CHAPTER 7

NUTS & SEEDS

Nuts and seeds have the ability to be either creamy or crunchy, which means they're super-versatile when it comes to their uses. Loaded with vitamins, minerals, protein, and healthy fats, they make an excellent snack on their own and add a nice crunch to salads and oatmeal. You can get inventive with them, too—such as turning soaked cashews into plant-based ice cream or soaked and dehydrated seeds into crackers or tortillas. And when they're ground, their crunchiness is transformed into decadent creaminess, making for delicious spreads and dressings.

Despite their health benefits, people are often afraid to eat them because of their higher calorie counts and fat content—but there's no need to avoid them. Study after study confirms that eating nuts shouldn't cause weight gain: In fact, they may even help you lose weight!

Nut & Seed Buzzwords

Nuts and seeds can be prepared in many ways, each of which affects their healthiness. Here are the terms you should know:

RAW

"Raw nuts" can mean two things. Most commonly, "raw" refers to nuts that have not been processed through roasting or heating. Nuts that have been processed—typically through sprouting followed by dehydration or low-temperature baking—are now also labeled "raw," as long as the temperature at which they were heated never exceeded 118°F (47.8°C). From a health perspective, the latter type of raw nuts—in which the nuts have been sprouted and dehydrated—are ideal. But raw nuts, in general, are preferable to roasted ones as high temperatures can oxidize their healthy natural oils.

SPROUTED

Sprouted nuts have been soaked and allowed to sprout—just like grains—which reduces their phytic acid, making them easier to digest and more nutritious. You can sprout them yourself or buy them pre-sprouted, in which case they'll also have been dehydrated or baked at a low temperature to increase shelf life and maintain their nutrients.

DRY ROASTED

Dry roasting is a process in which heat is applied to dry nuts and seeds without the use of oil. Dry-roasted nuts are preferable to roasted ones, but they're not as healthy as raw or sprouted nuts because this method subjects the delicate oils of the nuts to high heat.

ROASTED

Roasted nuts—the most common type found on supermarket shelves—are covered in oil and baked at high temperatures. They may even be fried, giving them that greasy, crispy, crunchy texture. Aside from the inferior, low-quality oils typically used on roasted nuts, the high temperatures may also alter and damage the delicate polyunsaturated fats naturally found in nuts, leading to oxidation and rancidity. Rancid oils are pro-inflammatory and carcinogenic, so roasted nuts are best avoided.

Benefits of Nuts & Seeds

Don't avoid nuts and seeds because of their high fat and calorie content. They offer a plethora of health benefits, including the following:

SUPPORT A HEALTHY WEIGHT

Multiple large and long-term studies have indicated that incorporating nuts into one's diet does not lead to weight gain as many people assume. Nuts have very high satiety value, which means they make you feel full. This, in turn, may lead to a lower overall calorie intake. Plus, our bodies don't absorb all the energy or fat from nuts. Between 5 and 20 percent of the calories and fat from nuts is not bioavailable to us. It passes through our digestive systems without being absorbed. Both factors contribute to nuts' role in maintaining a healthy body weight, despite their high calorie and fat content. In one study, Harvard researchers followed the diets of more than fifty thousand women over eight years and found that those who ate nuts two or more times a week were less likely to gain weight or become obese than those who rarely ate nuts. The results of this study suggest that incorporating nuts into the diet does not lead to greater weight gain and may help with weight control.

Some studies suggest that nuts may even assist weight loss. A small study published in the *International Journal of Obesity* found

◎ Myth Alert!

Myth: Fat makes you fat.

Fact: Fat is a necessary nutrient, crucial to every cell in the body, and also essential to a number of physiological functions, including hormone production, nutrient absorption, energy, protection of vital organs, and temperature regulation. The right types of fat, particularly whole-food plant-based fats such as those found in nuts, will not make you fat. Sugar is much more likely to make you fat.

So, don't be afraid of raw nuts, despite their high fat and calorie content. Studies show that regular consumption of raw nuts is associated with weight loss and lower body weight—not to mention longer, healthier lives with less risk of chronic disease.

that people who ate almonds daily lost more weight than those who ate a complex carb-rich diet with the same amount of calories. Researchers followed sixty five overweight or obese individuals over twenty-four weeks and found that those on the almond diet saw a decrease of 18 percent in weight and body mass index (BMI) compared with an 11 percent reduction in the non-almond dieters. Additionally, waist circumference in the almond group decreased by 14 percent, compared with 9 percent in the non-almond group.

SUPPORT HEART HEALTH

Thanks to their good fats, vitamin E, fiber, plant sterols, and the amino acid l-arginine, nuts support cardiovascular health. When consumed regularly, they may help lower bad LDL cholesterol, reduce the risk of blood clots, and improve the lining of your arteries.

SUPPORT BONE HEALTH

Nuts also support healthy bones, thanks to their magnesium content, which is needed for calcium absorption. Plus, nuts contain phytates, which may boost bone density and help prevent osteoporosis.

SUPPORT SKIN HEALTH

Nuts and seeds are a rich source of vitamin E, healthy fats—including anti-inflammatory omega-3s—and zinc, all of which support clear, supple skin.

Concerns About Nuts & Seeds

Nuts and seeds are a wonderful addition to your diet . . . but to get the most out of them, be sure to buy or prepare them properly. Here is what you need to know:

RAW VERSUS ROASTED

Nuts and seeds contain a large amount of oil, which can oxidize and go rancid quickly when heated to high temperatures, as with roasting. Rancid oils are pro-inflammatory and carcinogenic, so are best avoided. Plus, roasted nuts have added oils—such as canola, cottonseed, or other inferior oils—and salt. Instead, choose raw or soaked and dehydrated nuts and seeds. You can soak and dehydrate raw nuts and seeds yourself or find them presoaked and dehydrated at many health food stores and natural grocers. You can even find seasoned and flavored nuts prepared this way.

HARD TO DIGEST

Some people find nuts heavy or hard to digest, but there's an easy way to get around that. Soak nuts and seeds in lightly salted water overnight. This releases some of the enzyme inhibitors naturally present in the nuts or seeds that can cause digestive upset.

You can use soaked nuts for nut milks or other recipes, but if you won't be eating them right away, you must dehydrate or bake them at a low temperature to remove all the water and prevent molding.

ADDITIVES IN NUT BUTTERS

Nuts are expensive and some nut butter manufacturers cut costs by adding cheap fillers, such as palm oil or sugar syrups. Avoid them. When choosing nut butters, always check the ingredients list and only choose those that contain nuts alone—and, perhaps, salt.

PESTICIDES IN NUTS, NUT BUTTERS & SEEDS

Conventional nuts and seeds are subject to a wide array of pesticides, many of which may prove harmful to human health. Because nuts are high in fat, they may absorb pesticides and herbicides more easily than other less fatty foods so choose organic nuts to limit chemical exposure.

PASTEURIZED AMERICAN ALMONDS

Due to two separate salmonella outbreaks connected to California almond farms in the early 2000s, government regulations now mandate that all almonds grown or sold in the United States, Canada, or Mexico be pasteurized before being sold.

Two methods of pasteurization are generally used. Conventional American almonds are pasteurized with propylene oxide (PPO), which the EPA classifies as a probable human carcinogen. Organic American almonds are steam-pasteurized, which uses heat instead of chemicals to achieve the same result. To avoid toxic PPO, choose organic almonds. You can also purchase non-American almonds, such as Sicilian almonds, in some grocery stores or online. If you live near an almond

How to Soak Nuts & Seeds

Soaking raw nuts and seeds is a simple process, and it makes them more nutritious and easier to digest. Approximate nut and seed soak times are as follows:

Almonds: 8 to 12 hours
Brazil nuts: 2 to 3 hours
Cashews: 1 to 4 hours
Macadamias: 2 hours
Pecans: 6 hours
Pistachios: 8 hours
Pumpkin seeds: 8 hours
Sunflower seeds: 8 hours

1. **Soak raw nuts or seeds in salt water.** Fill a glass bowl with twice the amount of warm water than nuts or seeds. Add salt at a ratio of one-half teaspoon salt to one cup (235 ml) water. Let the salt dissolve before submerging the nuts or seeds. Cover the bowl with a clean kitchen towel or other breathable fabric and soak at room temperature according to the times listed.

2. **Drain and rinse.** Drain in a colander and rinse well. Always discard the soaking water as it contains all the stuff you don't want!

3. **Eat or process further.** You can eat the nuts and seeds as they are right away (you'll find them infinitely creamier!) or use them to make homemade nut milks, cheeses, dressings, or desserts. If not using immediately, dry them completely—dehydrate or bake them at the lowest temperature until they are completely dried throughout—to avoid mold. Baking time varies by nut or seed and oven temperature.

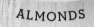

ALMONDS

CASHEWS

BRAZIL NUTS

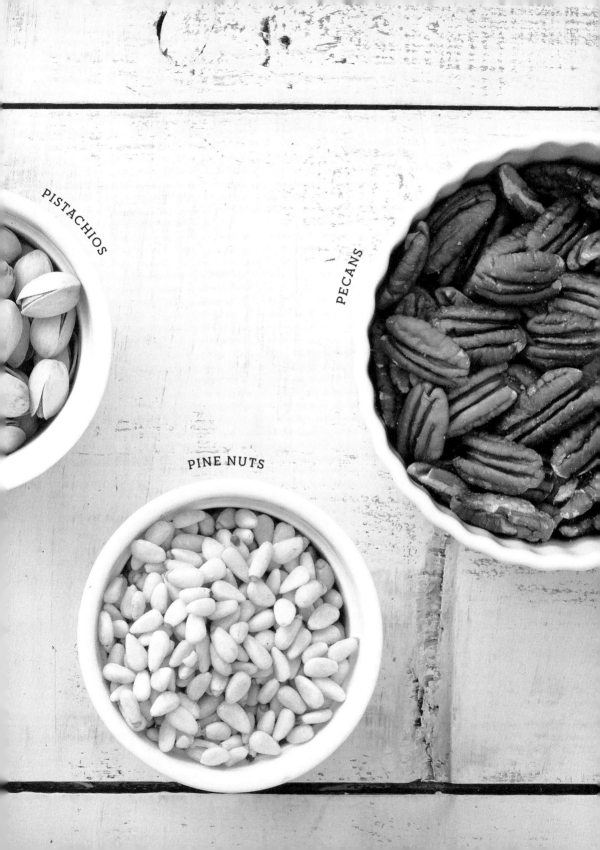

PISTACHIOS

PECANS

PINE NUTS

farm, you may be able to find nonpasteurized almonds at a local farmers' market. Almonds grown in Europe are not subject to the pasteurization mandate. Although no official legislation exists, almond growers in Australia typically pasteurize their almonds as well.

AFLATOXIN IN PEANUTS & TREE NUTS

Don't let their name fool you—peanuts aren't actually nuts, but legumes. Because they're grown underground, they're highly susceptible to aflatoxin, a liver-damaging toxin and potential carcinogen. Minute amounts of aflatoxin are found in the vast majority of peanut and peanut butter products, and, surprise, the grind-your-own peanut butter at grocery stores is usually the most heavily contaminated.

According to the International Food Policy Research Institute, consumption of aflatoxin may lead to liver damage, liver cancer, gastrointestinal dysfunction, immunosuppression, decreased appetite, and decreased reproductive function. In the United States, the government does limit the amount of aflatoxin allowed in human food products to 20 parts per billion (ppb), although other countries impose stricter standards based on health concerns. The European Union limits it to 10 ppb, and Canada and Australia limit it to 15 ppb. Research indicates that adult humans have a high tolerance for aflatoxin exposure and rarely succumb to poisoning by aflatoxin (aflatoxicosis), but children are more easily affected and their exposure to it can lead to stunted growth and delayed development.

Though some experts are concerned about chronic low-level exposure to this toxin, the FDA believes it poses little threat in the United States where it's consumed in relatively small amounts. But it's a bigger threat in developing countries, such as Kenya, where aflatoxin-susceptible products comprise a larger part of the diet and where outbreaks of aflatoxicosis, liver cancer, and death have resulted from the consumption of large amounts of tainted foods. However, there have been no known outbreaks of aflatoxicosis in the United States.

If you eat peanuts and peanut butter, eat them in small amounts and consider pairing them with veggies such as celery, carrots, or greens. At least one study shows that eating peanut butter with vegetables, particularly chlorophyll-rich greens, inhibits aflatoxin's carcinogenic affects.

Though peanuts are the most aflaxotin-susceptible "nut" in the United States, aflatoxins can also be found in corn and corn products, cottonseed, milk, and tree nuts such as almonds, Brazil nuts, pecans, pistachios, and walnuts. Contamination can occur, but tree nuts are much less susceptible to it than peanuts.

Ingesting aflatoxin may not be detrimental when consumed irregularly and in small quantities, but you can avoid it by replacing peanut butter with almond, sunflower, or cashew butter and peanuts with any other nuts or seeds.

⊗ Money-Saving Tip

Buy bulk goods online. It's easy to find organic nuts (and grains and legumes, too) online, sometimes at cheaper prices than grocery stores offer.

Types of Nuts & Nut Butters

You can choose from many different nuts and nut butters, each offering a different nutrient and flavor profile. Here are the most common:

ALMONDS

Almonds are an excellent source of vitamin E. One ounce (28 g) provides 37 percent of your recommended DV—which supports skin, eye, cardiac, and immune system health. They also contain healthy monounsaturated fats, which are associated with heart health and lower cholesterol. Avoid almonds that look dusty—they're past their prime. Choose organic because nonorganic almonds are pasteurized with the chemical PPO, which the EPA classifies as a probable human carcinogen.

BRAZIL NUTS

Just one Brazil nut contains more than 100 percent of your DV of selenium, a powerful antioxidant which plays a role in immunity, aids the metabolism, and may help protect against cancer.

CASHEWS

Typically considered a nut, cashews are actually a seed. Cashews are a great source of energy and support skin, bone, and brain health. One ounce (28 g) contains 10 percent of your iron needs (for energy); 11 percent of zinc (for immune health); 20 percent of magnesium (which calms nerves and anxiety); and 23 percent of manganese (for bone health). Cashew butter is decadently rich and creamy, making it a great base for ice creams and other healthier desserts.

HAZELNUTS

Hazelnuts are rich in vitamins and minerals that support skin, heart, and bone health, including manganese, magnesium, iron, and copper as well as vitamin E.

MACADAMIA NUTS

Rich, buttery macadamias are an excellent source of monounsaturated fats, which support heart health. They also provide a hefty dose of manganese (58 percent of your DV per ounce, or 28 g) and vitamin B_1 or thiamin, a nutrient that supports energy levels and healthy metabolism (delivering 22 percent DV per ounce, or 28 g).

PINE NUTS

Like cashews, pine nuts are also seeds. They contain anti-aging compounds, support heart health, and studies suggest they may even suppress appetite. They also contain lutein, which is vital to eye health, and minerals needed to maintain energy levels, including magnesium and iron.

PISTACHIOS

Nutrient-dense pistachios are loaded with antioxidants that support heart health, a healthy body weight, and balanced blood sugar. At four calories per nut, they're the least calorie-dense of all nuts. Coupled with the fact that eating them from the shell automatically makes you eat them slowly, they make a great snack choice!

PEANUTS

Peanuts provide a variety of minerals and vitamins. However, as discussed on page 152, peanuts can contain aflatoxin, which is best avoided. You can get the same vitamins and minerals that peanuts offer—plus a healthier fatty acid profile—from other nuts and seeds, so consider switching from peanut butter to almond butter, cashew butter, or sunflower butter.

PECANS

At nearly three grams of fiber per ounce (28 g), pecans support digestive and heart health. One ounce (28 g) also provides 8 percent of your DV of zinc, which promotes clear skin and a strong immune

Minerals

Nuts are a great source of minerals, which are nutrients you need on a daily basis for your body to function properly. Though each mineral serves multiple purposes, here's a brief summary of each mineral's best-known benefits.

MAJOR MINERALS

Calcium: supports bone health, aids in muscle contraction, and helps blood clot

Chloride: helps maintain the proper balance of bodily fluids

Magnesium: supports bone health, aids in muscle and nerve function, and keeps heart rhythm steady; a lack of magnesium may trigger migraines and PMS

Phosphorus: promotes bone health and is important for metabolism and cognitive function

Potassium: helps maintain normal blood pressure and supports kidney health

Sodium: important for maintaining the proper balance of bodily fluids, regulating blood pressure, and supporting the adrenal glands

Sulfur: promotes hair, skin, nail, and muscle health

TRACE MINERALS

Chromium: plays a key role in the regulation of blood sugar

Copper: builds tissue, maintains blood volume, and aids in energy production

Fluoride: strengthens bones and prevents tooth decay

Iodine: supports proper thyroid function

Iron: important for energy and helps transport oxygen throughout the body

Manganese: plays a role in collagen production and supports skin health; low levels may contribute to bone malformation and even infertility

Molybdenum: aids in metabolism of fats and carbohydrates

Selenium: promotes cognitive function, a healthy immune system, and fertility

Zinc: supports healthy skin, a strong immune system, learning and memory capacity, and male fertility; eating zinc-rich foods when you have a cold or flu may shorten the duration and severity of it

system. As one of the most antioxidant-rich nuts, pecans may help prevent plaque formation in the arteries.

WALNUTS

Walnuts contain a healthy dose of anti-inflammatory omega-3s, which support skin and brain health. They also contain antioxidants that support heart health by reducing high blood pressure and helping the body deal with stress. Plus, animal studies have shown promising results for potential anti-tumor and anticancer effects.

Types of Seeds & Seed Butters

Beyond offering a little crunch to any dish, seeds provide a variety of nutrients and health benefits. They may be small, but they're mighty! Here are some of the most common:

CHIA SEEDS

Chia seeds are extremely high in anti-inflammatory omega-3s, which has helped them earn their "superfood" status (one ounce, or 28 g, contains nearly ten times the recommended DV). They're high in fiber (nearly 11 g per ounce, or 42 percent of your DV), which keeps you full and encourages regularity. They're an excellent source of sustainable, long-lasting energy, so throw them into your morning smoothie to keep hunger pangs at bay for hours. They're also a complete protein, which is particularly important if you're following a plant-based diet.

FLAXSEED

Another anti-inflammatory all-star, flaxseed is loaded with omega-3s. Plus it's high in fiber and protein as well as lignans, a phytochemical associated with decreased cancer risk. Add it to oatmeal, smoothies, rice, and salads.

It's important to note, though, our bodies can't absorb all the healthy goodness of flaxseed when it's whole. To reap its benefits, grind flax before eating it. Ideally, buy whole flaxseed and grind it in a clean coffee or spice grinder just before consuming it. If that's not an option, you can buy milled flaxseed, which is preground. Just remember to refrigerate it and use it quickly; it goes rancid faster when it's ground.

HEMP SEEDS

Hemp seeds are an excellent source of complete plant-based protein at more than ten grams per ounce (28 g). The same amount contains more than seven grams of anti-inflammatory omega-3s. Throw an ounce (about three tablespoons, or 28 g) of hemp seeds into your smoothie instead of protein powder or toss the seeds on breakfast bowls or salads.

❗ Expert Tip

The trick to unlocking chia seeds' incredibly cleansing fiber power is soaking them. They absorb up to ten times their weight in water and will form a gel that keeps you satiated for hours. Simply add one tablespoon (13 g) chia seeds to 1 cup (235 ml) water (or other liquid such as juice) and let it sit for at least ten minutes. The seeds become suspended throughout the liquid, and though they may look weird, they won't change the liquid's taste—especially when blended into a smoothie. "Hydrated" chia is easier to digest than dry chia, so always soak it before consuming it.

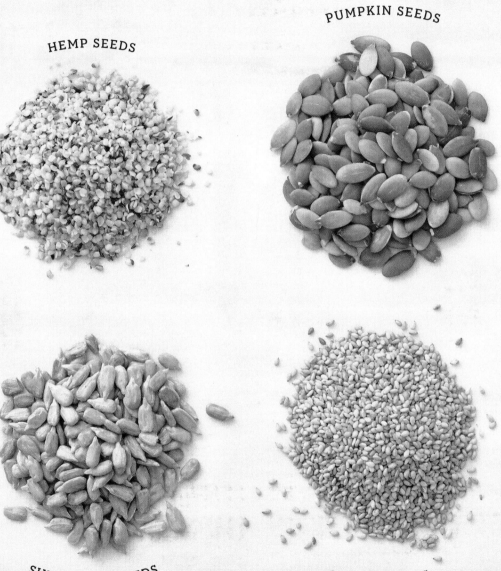

HEMP SEEDS

PUMPKIN SEEDS

SUNFLOWER SEEDS

SESAME SEEDS

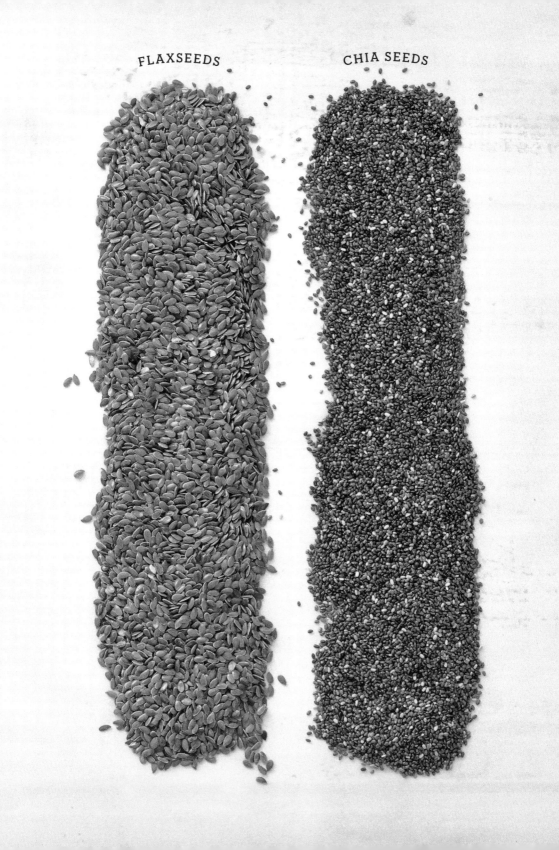

FLAXSEEDS   CHIA SEEDS

PUMPKIN SEEDS

Pumpkin seeds are mineral-rich powerhouses. A quarter cup (40 g) contains 23 percent of the recommended DV of zinc, which promotes a strong immune system and clear skin, as well as 48 percent DV of magnesium, which can help eliminate headaches and migraines. They also exhibit antibacterial and antiparasitic properties.

SESAME SEEDS

Sesame seeds do more than just offer a nutty crunch or Asian twist to your dishes. They also provide a plethora of minerals, including copper, calcium, and magnesium. Sprinkle them on a veggie stir-fry, salads, oatmeal, or homemade crackers.

Sesame seed butter is called tahini and is a key ingredient in hummus. You can use it to make a creamy salad dressing (simply whisk it with double the amount of water and a pinch of salt), or pair it with honey to make halva, a simple Middle Eastern dessert.

SUNFLOWER SEEDS

Sunflower seeds are an excellent source of B vitamins, vitamin E, copper, and other minerals. They provide anti-inflammatory benefits, which may offer relief for arthritis and asthma sufferers. They support heart health and because they are high in magnesium, may help prevent migraines.

Sunflower seed butter is another great alternative to peanut butter and can be used in dressings and desserts.

How to Choose & Store Nuts & Seeds

- Choose raw or soaked and dehydrated nuts and seeds.

- Choose pure nut butters, free of palm oil and sweeteners.

- Choose organic almonds to avoid PPO, a probable human carcinogen.

- Choose organic for other types of nuts when you can to limit pesticide exposure.

- Try healthier alternatives to peanuts. To avoid aflatoxin, choose other nuts, seeds, or their butters as replacements for peanuts and peanut butter.

STORE WISELY

Because nuts and seeds contain healthy oils, they will go rancid in time, making them unhealthy. It's best to refrigerate nuts, seeds, and opened jars of nut and seed butters to prolong shelf life and protect them from heat or light. It's a good idea to buy smaller portions—only what you'll consume in a month or so—to ensure freshness.

❶ Expert Tip

Suggested Serving Size Guidelines for Nuts and Seeds	
Serving size:	One handful of nuts or seeds (about one ounce or 28 g); one tablespoon (16 g) nut butter
Servings per day:	One to three
Frequency per week:	Every day, or at least two or more times per week

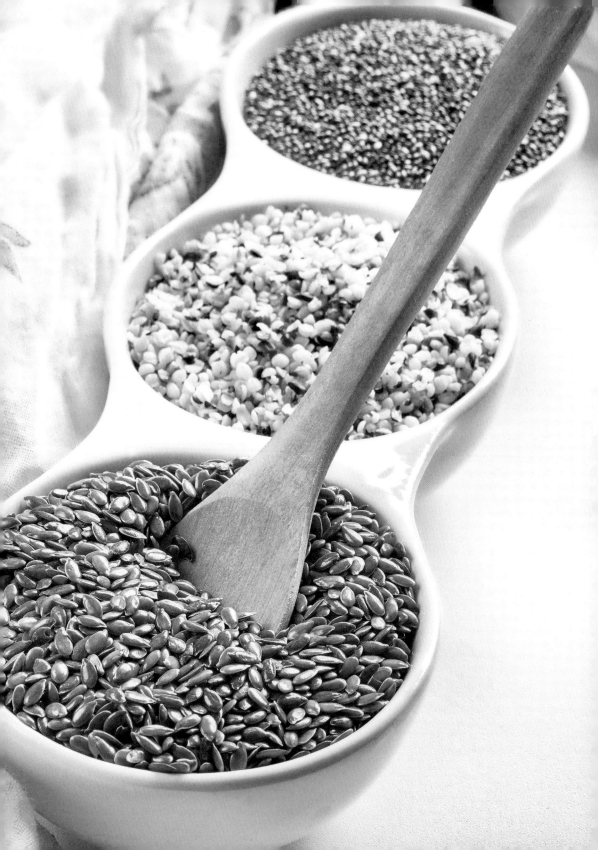

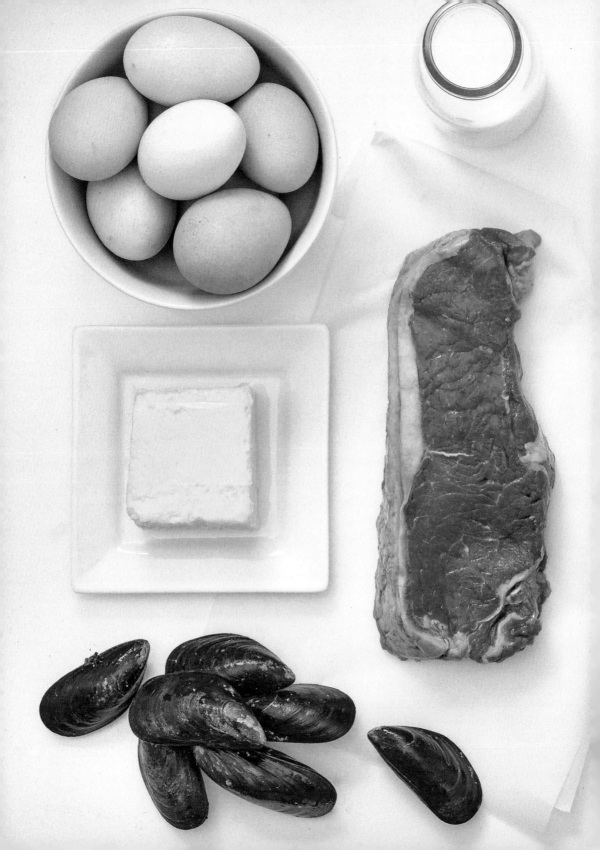

PART III

ANIMAL-BASED WHOLE FOODS

Shopping for the Healthiest Options. For those who eat a typical Western diet, it's not a meal without meat, and not a day goes by without some form of dairy, such as milk or cheese. You'll learn in the coming chapters that one of the best things we can do for our health is to not only limit our consumption of animal products, but choose the highest quality when we do consume them. This section teaches you how to do just that.

CHAPTER 8

MEAT & POULTRY

For people in many parts of the world (such as the United States, Australia, the United Kingdom, and much of Europe), it's not a meal without meat. According to research by the Organization for Economic Cooperation and Development, while the global average per capita meat consumption is 75 pounds (34 kg) annually, Americans and Australians are practically tied in first place for the highest consumption, at just less than 200 pounds (91 kg) of meat per person, per year. New Zealand (161 lb, or 73 kg), Canada (152 lb, or 69 kg), and Europe (143 lb, or 65 kg) aren't far behind.

In recent years, however, books such as *The China Study* and documentaries such as *Forks Over Knives* have exposed some serious health concerns of a diet high in animal products. Overall meat consumption, in the United States, at least, is slowly declining. This is particularly true for consumption of red meat. Based on USDA data, meat consumption peaked in 2004, with average per capita consumption estimated at 170 pounds (77 kg). By 2013, that number dropped to about 155 pounds (70 kg).

Still Americans overall eat more than the recommended amount of meat. The current USDA guidelines suggest no more than 3 to 4 ounces (85 to 115 g) per day (and some nutrition experts think that's too much). But many people routinely consume double that amount.

As you'll learn in this chapter, compelling research supports cutting back on meat and animal products because higher intake of these products is associated with higher risk of many common diseases, including cancers. This isn't to say you have to eschew all animal products for ideal health. Small amounts of high-quality animal products can fit into a healthy diet. After educating yourself on the benefits and concerns outlined in this chapter, the choice is yours. Know you can easily (and more economically!) satisfy at least some, or even all, of your protein needs through plant-based foods, as discussed in chapter 6—but if you choose to consume meat, the two most important factors to consider are *quality* and *amount*. It pays to be a conscious consumer—especially at the butcher's counter.

Meat & Poultry Buzzwords

When buying meat and poultry, from a health perspective, *quality* is the most important factor to consider. Following are the terms that will help you evaluate the quality of any type of meat:

RED MEAT

Red meat is meat that comes from a mammal: generally, beef, veal, pork, lamb, mutton, and goat. The World Health Organization classifies red meat as a probable human carcinogen, so you may want to consume it sparingly.

POULTRY

Poultry is meat from a bird, such as chicken or turkey.

WHITE MEAT

White meat comes from poultry, so poultry is sometimes referred to as white meat. More specifically, it refers to the lighter-colored meat in the carcass (breast meat, for example) and excludes the darker meat in the leg or thigh.

PROCESSED MEAT

Processed meat is any meat transformed through salting, curing, fermentation, smoking, or other processes to enhance flavor or improve preservation. This includes hot dogs, sausages, smoked meats, ham, corned beef, beef jerky, and canned meats. The World Health Organization has classified processed meat as a human carcinogen, so it's best avoided or consumed in limited amounts.

MEAT

Meat refers to both red and white meat.

The following buzzwords apply to all meat products, including red meat and poultry, but not fish or seafood, discussed in chapter 9.

ORGANIC

Organic meat comes from animals that have not been given artificial growth hormones or antibiotics, which may be the most important reason to choose organic meat—always. Certain hormones have been linked to cancer, and the frequent consumption of antibiotics has been linked to antibiotic resistance. Additionally, with organic meat, the animal's feed is certified organic, and the animal must have outdoor access.

KOSHER

While a kosher symbol signifies food that satisfies Jewish law, it also symbolizes higher-quality standards, in general—and that means you may want to purchase kosher animal products, regardless of your religion. The way that Kosher meats are prepared may reduce the likelihood of spreading foodborne illness and the way the animal is slaughtered is believed to be the least painful.

Beef Buzzwords

Because not all buzzwords apply to all types of meat or have the same meaning in all situations, I've broken them down here by type to help you easily see what to look for, depending on what you're purchasing.

PASTURE RAISED

This is a term used for cattle that spent a significant amount of time outdoors, on pasture, as opposed to in the small, confined indoor areas typical of most factory farms. Unlike grass-fed cows, which eat only their natural diet of grass, pasture-raised cows may also receive supplemental organic grains, both during the grazing season and in the winter months. (This is a good beef choice.)

GRASS FED

Grass-fed beef is from animals fed their natural diet of grass instead of grains.

This leads to healthier animals and healthier meat. These animals should have continuous access to pasture during growing season—although an animal that was both grass-fed and raised without confinement is ideal. (This is a better beef choice.)

FOOD ALLIANCE CERTIFIED GRASS-FED

This term ensures the animal was raised both without confinement and fed a natural diet of grass. Alternatively, look for meat that's labeled both pasture raised and grass fed.

Poultry Buzzwords

Here are poultry-specific terms to help guide your shopping.

CAGE FREE

All poultry raised for meat is cage free, so this term on meat packaging doesn't have much relevance (but it does have meaning for eggs, see chapter 10). Cage free indicates the animal was not confined to a small battery cage, but does not necessarily mean it was allowed outside or given ample space to move around.

◎ **Myth Alert!**

Myth: You need to eat meat for protein.

Fact: Meat does contain protein but it's not the only source of it. Quinoa, buckwheat, soy, beans, lentils, grains, nuts, seeds, and even fruits and vegetables all contain protein. And it's entirely possible to get adequate protein strictly from plants, if you choose to do so. It may take a little more planning, but it's doable. (For more on plant protein, see chapter 6.)

FREE RANGE, FREE ROAMING

This is a term used for poultry to indicate it was allowed some freedom of movement outside. However, because "outside" is not a legally defined term, this could mean the animal spends five minutes outside daily, and this time doesn't have to be spent on pasture—it could be a concrete parking lot. (This is a better poultry choice.)

PASTURE RAISED

This indicates the animal spent a significant amount of time in the outdoors, on pasture, and spends only the night indoors. This is the most natural lifestyle and leads to the healthiest poultry. (This is the best poultry choice.)

Lamb Buzzwords

Following are the buzzwords you need to keep in mind when selecting lamb.

GRASS FED

Grass-fed lamb is from animals fed their natural diet of grass instead of grains. This leads to healthier animals and healthier meat. These animals should have continuous access to pasture during growing season—although an animal that was both grass-fed and raised without confinement is ideal. (This is a better lamb choice.)

PASTURE RAISED

This term indicates the animal spent a significant amount of its time outdoors, foraging for a natural diet on the pasture, as opposed to indoors. (This is the best choice.)

Pork & Goat Buzzwords

The following will help guide your pork and goat meat purchases.

PASTURE RAISED

This is a term used to indicate the animal spent a significant amount of its time outdoors, foraging for a natural diet on the pasture, as opposed to indoors.

Pigs and goats don't naturally eat grass, so while you may see pork and goat meat labeled "grass fed," it's not important.

Benefits of Meat & Poultry

Meat and poultry are best known for adding protein to our diets, but they also supply certain critical nutrients—and flavor. Here are some benefits of meat and poultry:

COMPLETE PROTEIN

All animal products are complete proteins, meaning, as we've seen previously, they contain all the essential amino acids we need to consume each day.

VITAMIN B$_{12}$

B$_{12}$ is a critical nutrient found almost exclusively in animal-based foods. It plays a key role in normal brain and nervous system function. If you're vegan or following a plant-based diet, supplementation with B$_{12}$ is necessary.

FLAVOR

Many people simply think meat tastes good. And while you don't necessarily need to forgo it completely for vibrant health, it's wise to think of meat as a condiment or side dish instead of the main event. For optimum health, use meat to flavor your dishes and allow vegetables to be the stars.

PROVIDES IRON

Red meat and poultry are good sources of iron. Iron helps your body produce red blood cells which transport oxygen to different parts of the body. Iron from animal products, called, heme iron, is absorbed more readily than the non-heme iron found in plant-based foods.

Concerns About Meat & Poultry

Consuming large amounts of meat and poultry is cause for concern, as is the way these animals are raised on factory farms. Here is what you should know:

HORMONES & ANTIBIOTICS

The use of hormones and antibiotics in meat brings up significant concerns. Factory-farmed animals are raised in unnatural conditions and routinely given synthetic hormones and antibiotics, which results in meat that could pose a serious risk to human health. Since 1989, the European Union (EU) has refused to import meat from animals administered synthetic hormones (including those from the United States) because of the potential health risks; some of the hormones used are known or suspected carcinogens linked to breast and reproductive cancers. (Organic meat, which is free of added hormones, was not affected by the ban.) One of the six hormones banned in the EU, yet approved and used in the United States, is estradiol-17β, classified as a human carcinogen by the U.S. National Toxicology Program.

The Centers for Disease Control and Prevention has warned that the intake of meat from antibiotic-fed animals could lead to antibiotic-resistant infections in humans. Globally, these types of infections kill an estimated 700,000 people each year. The death toll is expected to rise significantly if we continue the way we are going. The UK's chief medical officer, Dame Sally Davies, ranked

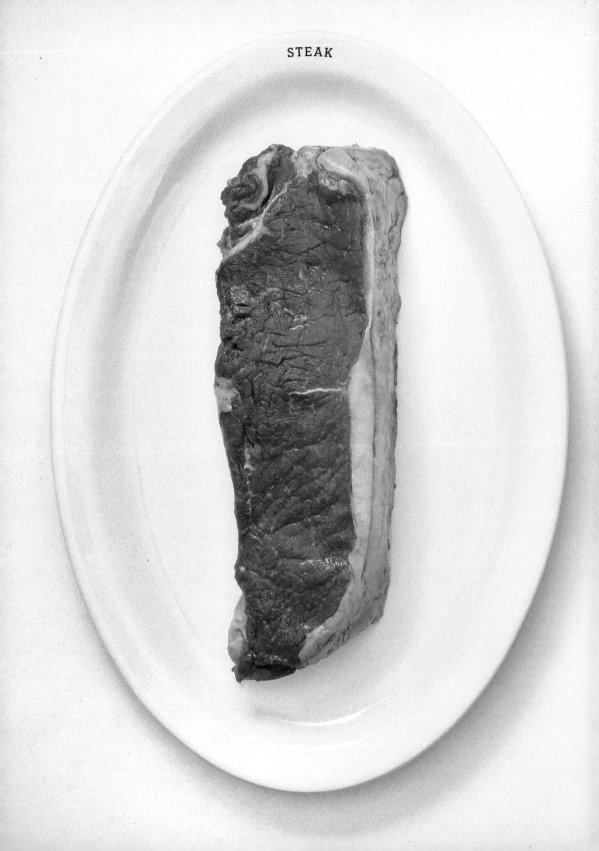

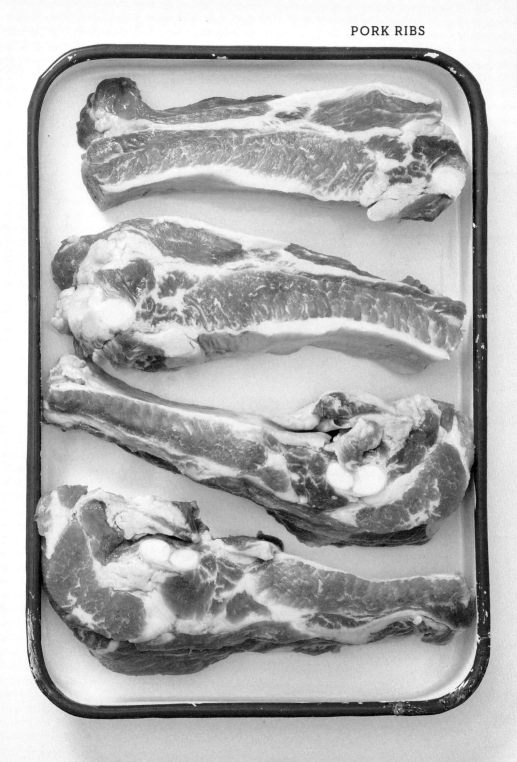

antibiotic-resistant bacteria as serious a threat to society as climate change. "Antimicrobial resistance poses a catastrophic threat. If we don't act now, any one of us could go into a hospital in twenty years for minor surgery and die because of an ordinary infection that can't be treated by antibiotics. Routine operations like hip replacements or organ transplants could be deadly because of the risk of infection." Choose organic meat to avoid both synthetic hormones and antibiotics.

INCREASED RISK OF HEART DISEASE & CANCER

Heart disease is the number one killer worldwide, claiming more than six hundred thousand people each year in the United States alone, which accounts for one in four deaths. Thanks to decades of meticulous studies by cardiologist Dean Ornish, M.D., heart disease has been scientifically proven to be avoidable—and even reversible—by replacing the bulk of animal-based foods with plant-based foods and by managing stress, exercising, and seeking a support network.

Research conducted at Harvard's School of Public Health has found that even eating small amounts of red meat is linked to an increased risk of heart disease and stroke. Replacing one serving of red meat per day with poultry, fish, nuts, or beans lowered that risk. Processed meat in particular—such as bacon or hot dogs—was even more strongly linked to increased cardiovascular disease risk: Just one and a half ounces (42 g) daily increases your risk by 20 percent.

A wide and growing body of evidence suggests limiting overall meat intake and to choose fish, chicken, and plant-based proteins over red meat and processed meat.

❗ Expert Tip

Limiting animal product consumption and increasing vegetable intake lowers your risk for many chronic illnesses, including heart disease and colon cancer, studies show. Although the *2015–2020 Dietary Guidelines for Americans* suggests limiting meat, poultry, and egg intake to about six to eight 3- to 4-ounce (85 to 113 g) servings per week, in my opinion, consuming meat four to five meals per week is sufficient. The rest of your meals should contain protein from plant-based sources such as quinoa, beans, and lentils, or seafood (up to twice a week).

BACTERIAL CONTAMINATION

Kosher certification on meat products signifies the highest slaughtering standards, so it's less likely to be contaminated with fecal matter. To limit or avoid cross-contamination, choose kosher meats.

NITRATES & NITRITES IN PROCESSED MEATS

Deli meats, hot dogs, sausages, and other processed meats typically contain nitrates and nitrites, which are classified as "probable human carcinogens" by the International Agency for Research on Cancer. So, limit or avoid processed meats and when you do have them, look for brands that don't contain nitrates or nitrites.

ENVIRONMENTAL POLLUTION & CLIMATE CHANGE

In 2013 a report by the United Nations Food and Agriculture Organization found that the meat and dairy industries contribute more to greenhouse gas emissions—believed to be contributing to climate change and the melting of our ice caps—than the entire transportation industry. Producing just one half pound (225 g) of hamburger meat releases as much greenhouse gas into the atmosphere as driving a 3,000 pound (1,361 kg) car for nearly 10 miles (16 km). Rajendra Pachauri, Ph.D., chair of the United Nations Intergovernmental Panel on Climate Change, has suggested that if everyone were to forgo meat just one day a week, we could make a significant positive impact on reducing greenhouse gases.

Safe Shopping & Storage Tips for Meat & Poultry

At the grocery store, always pick up meat or poultry last, so it doesn't get warm sitting in your cart. Additionally:

- Choose packages with the latest expiration date: This indicates it's freshest.

- Never choose torn or leaking packages.

- Place raw meat or poultry in plastic bags and tie them to prevent

❗ Expert Tip

Suggested Serving Size Guidelines for Meat	
Serving size:	Four ounces (115 g), about the size of an iPhone 6
Servings per day:	None to one
Frequency per week:	Four to five meals per week

❗ Expert Tip

Buying & Selecting Meat

To ensure you always get the highest quality meat products, shop the following:

- Farmers' markets
- Health food stores
- Direct from small local farms

Or check out www.eatwild.com/products/index.html to find producers in your area.
When purchasing meat, consider the following:

- Choose organic and kosher.
- For beef and lamb, always choose grass fed. Food Alliance Certified Grass-Fed is the highest third-party stamp of approval for beef.
- For chicken and turkey, opt for pasture raised. Free range varieties are your next best option.
- Avoid processed meats that contain nitrites and nitrates.

cross-contaminations; otherwise, blood or juices may leak onto other foods.

- Put meat or poultry on ice in a cooler bag if it takes you longer than thirty minutes to travel home.

- Store meat on the refrigerator's bottom shelf in a closed plastic bag to prevent blood or juices from leaking onto other foods.

- Cook or freeze poultry, ground meat, and organ meat within two days of purchase and cook or freeze beef, veal, lamb, or pork within three to five days.

CHAPTER 9

SEAFOOD

Seafood can be a delicious way to add protein and B vitamins to your plate. It's also an important source of essential omega-3 fatty acids. And with dozens of different types of fish and other seafood on the market, you're bound to find at least one you like.

As with meat, though, the quality of seafood should be your first concern, especially if you consume it regularly. Why? Well, as the demand for fish has increased, the ways in which we source it have changed. While some fishermen still go out on open waters with a pole and line, they are few and far between. Instead, like cattle and other livestock, much of our fish is farmed, so there are concerns. And, whether it's farmed or wild, mercury and PCB contamination are additional concerns when it comes to seafood. This chapter shows you how to choose seafood wisely.

Seafood Buzzwords

When choosing seafood, quality is key. Learn the meaning behind these common terms to make the best choices.

FARM RAISED

Farmed fish can be raised either in a tank or within a net placed in a natural body of water. These fish are typically vaccinated (either through injection, immersion in water containing diluted vaccine, or through feed) and fed

hormones and antibiotics because the close quarters in which they live breed disease. Certain varieties are also subject to pesticide use. Farming fish in natural water is destructive to the ecosystem outside of the net, and nearby wild fish populations are sometimes wiped out by disease as a result.

ORGANIC

The term "organic" farmed fish is sort of an oxymoron. At the time of writing, the USDA has not yet clearly defined the term "organic" for seafood, so this label may not mean much. The USDA is working on a standard definition, but many organic advocates are not thrilled about this because for all other organic meat, the animals must be fed an organic diet to meet organic standards. But farmed fish labeled "organic" are fed wild fish, which are not necessarily up to organic standards.

WILD

Grocery store fish labeled "wild" are not truly wild; they're raised in wild fisheries within rivers, lakes, and oceans. They are different, though, from farmed fish in that they're not treated with antibiotics, hormones, pesticides, or vaccines. Wild fish are a better choice than farmed. (This is a good seafood choice.)

LINE-CAUGHT

Line-caught fish are caught by towing a line with multiple baited hooks—sometimes thousands of hooks—behind a slow-moving boat. Line-caught fish are a better choice than wild.

POLE-CAUGHT/POLE AND LINE

Pole and line fishing are probably what you imagine when you think of fishing: One hook one line; one fisherman catching one fish at a time. From a health perspective, pole-caught fish is on par with line-caught because they are both truly wild. However, pole-caught is the most socially and environmentally responsible way of fishing.

Benefits of Seafood

Seafood is a good source of a few key nutrients, such as essential omega-3 fatty acids and iodine, not readily found in other foods, making it a great addition to a healthy diet. Here are some benefits:

OMEGA-3

Fish are one of the most abundant sources of essential omega-3 fatty acids, which must be consumed through the diet for good health. Fish have two types of omega-3s—EPA and DHA—which are required for proper brain and cardiovascular function.

B VITAMINS

In general, fish are a good source of B vitamins, including B_{12}. All B vitamins play important roles in cell metabolism, helping you get energy from the food you eat. B vitamins are also needed for red blood cell formation.

IODINE

Iodine is a mineral your body needs to make thyroid hormones, which control metabolism and many other bodily functions. Fish are a great source of iodine. Other food sources include seaweed, sea vegetables, and eggs.

COMPLETE PROTEIN

Fish are a complete protein as they contain all essential amino acids our bodies need to consume each day.

Concerns About Seafood

Though fish can be a healthy part of your diet, the way we source fish raises some concerns. Here is what you should know:

ANTIBIOTICS

Fish are typically raised in overcrowded tanks or pens, which are breeding grounds for viruses, diseases, and parasites. They also require large amounts of space, so the close quarters often cause them to develop stress and nervous disorders. As such, they are vaccinated or routinely receive antibiotics that can make it on to your plate. Vaccinations can be given either through injection, immersion (putting fish in vaccine-treated water for a period of time), or orally through feed. As with meat, the use of antibiotics can lead to antibiotic-resistant bacteria.

In the United States, a "waiting period" exists during which fish are taken off the antibiotics for thirty to 180 days to reduce or remove the drugs from their systems before

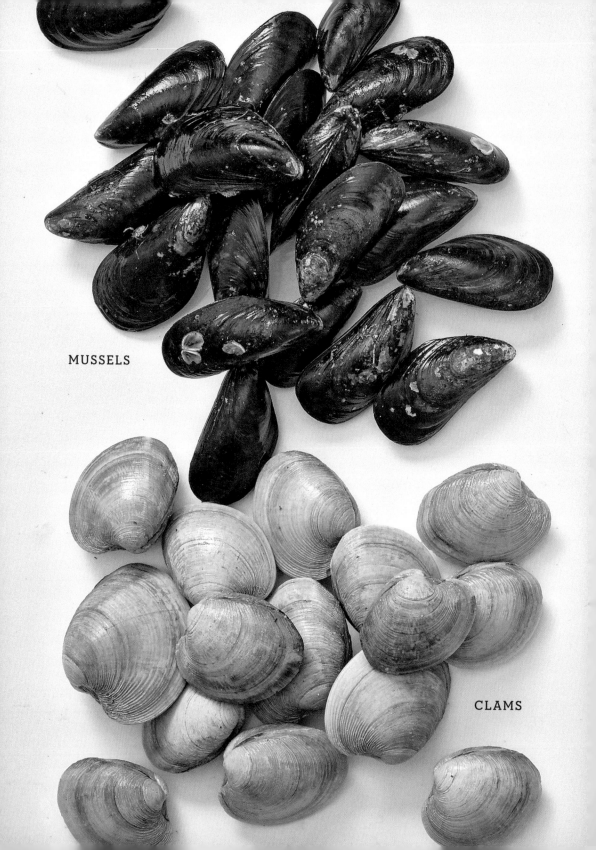

MUSSELS

CLAMS

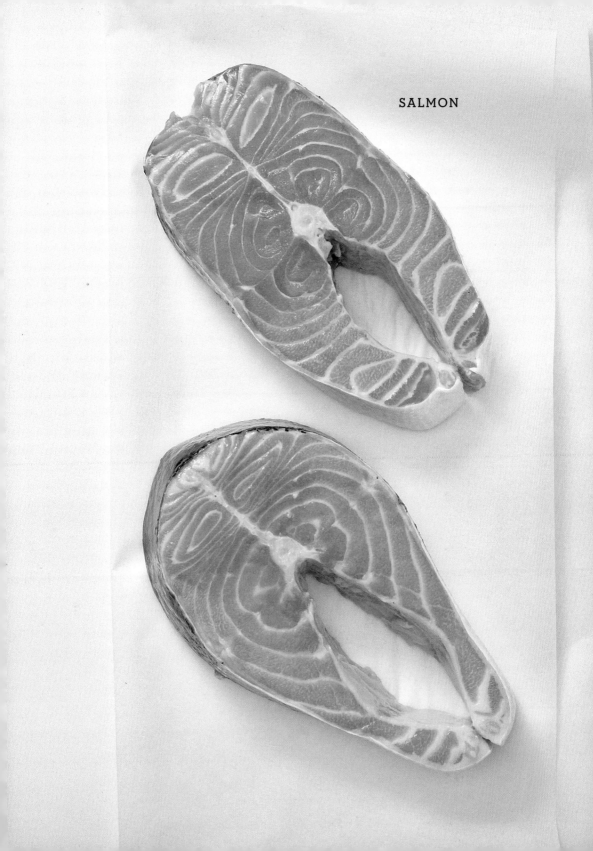

SALMON

Mercury Levels of Fish

Least Mercury	Moderate Mercury *Eat six servings or fewer per month*	High Mercury *Eat three servings or fewer per month*
Anchovies	Bass (striped, black)	Bluefish
Butterfish	Carp	Grouper*
Catfish	Cod (Alaskan)	Mackerel (Spanish, gulf)
Clam	Croaker (white Pacific)	Sea bass (Chilean)
Crab (domestic)*	Halibut (Atlantic*, Pacific)	Tuna (canned albacore*, yellowfin*)
Crawfish/crayfish	Jacksmelt (silverside)	
Croaker (Atlantic)	Lobster	
Flounder	Mahimahi*	
Haddock (Atlantic)*	Monkfish	
Hake	Perch (freshwater)	
Herring	Sablefish	
Mackerel (North Atlantic, Chub)	Skate	
Mullet	Snapper	
Oyster	Tuna (canned chunk light*, skipjack*)	
Perch (ocean)	Weakfish (sea trout)	
Plaice		
Pollock		
Salmon (canned, Alaskan, Atlantic*)		
Sardine		
Scallop		
Shad (American)		
Shrimp		
Sole (Pacific)		
Squid (calamari)		
Tilapia		
Trout (freshwater)		
Whitefish		
Whiting		

Source: Mercury level recommendations taken from the U.S. Natural Resources Defense Council. Sustainability taken from the Monterey Bay Aquarium Seafood Watch.
*Indicates the species is not sustainable and is overfished. Best choices are those with low to moderate mercury levels, with no accompanying asterisk.

Highest Mercury	Least Sustainable
Avoid eating	
Mackerel (king)	Cod (Atlantic, Canada, and U.S.)
Marlin	Crab (Atlantic rock and Jonah, U.S.)
Orange roughy*	Crab (canned, imported)
Shark*	Crab, red king (Russia)
Swordfish	Haddock (Gulf of Maine)
Tilefish	Halibut (Atlantic, U.S.)
Tuna* (bigeye, ahi)	Mahimahi (imported)
	Orange roughy
	Salmon (farmed)
	Sardines (Atlantic, Mediterranean)
	Shark
	Shrimp (imported)
	Squid (imported, U.S. okay)
	Swordfish (imported longline)
	Tuna, albacore (except U.S. troll, pole & line, and longline); bluefin; and skipjack (imported purse seine)
	Tuna, yellowfin (except troll, pole & line, and HI longline)

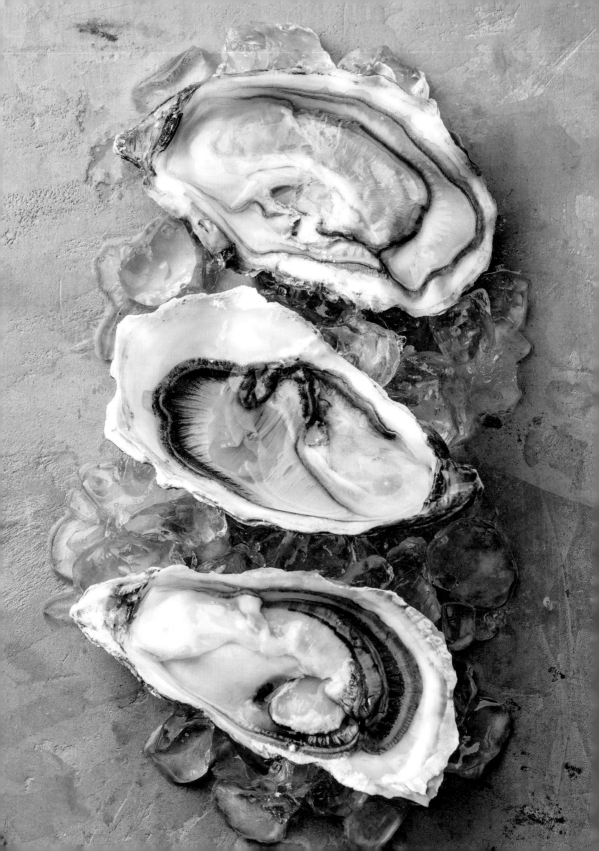

being sold. Some antibiotics used in South American fisheries are banned in the United States—yet the fish that are fed them can end up in American grocery stores. Wild fish, on the other hand, are not given antibiotics.

PESTICIDES

Pesticide use is a concern for certain farmed fish. Farming fish damages the ecosystem, making the fish—particularly farmed salmon—more susceptible to parasites, such as sea lice. If they're not removed, sea lice can be deadly to fish. Therefore, pesticides are administered, either via immersion or orally, to kill the sea lice—and again, these pesticides may end up to some extent on your plate.

Having just looked at risks specific to farmed fish, the following concerns are applicable to *all* fish.

MERCURY & PCBs

Unfortunately, factories and acid rain have contaminated most, if not all, of our bodies of water with mercury (a heavy metal that is a neurotoxin that interferes with the brain and nervous system) and PCBs (polychlorinated biphenyl, a known endocrine disruptor and a suspected human carcinogen). Although everyone should be concerned about these chemicals, women who are pregnant or trying to become pregnant especially should avoid PCB exposure as it can cause significant neurological and motor control problems, including lowered IQ, in unborn children.

Most, if not all, fish contain traces of these chemicals, but the exact amounts depend on how and where the fish were raised. Studies show that farmed fish tend to have higher levels of PCBs. For example, a report published by the Environmental Working Group found

❗ Expert Tip

Here's a simple trick to ordering fish that is least contaminated with mercury or PCBs: *Choose fish the size of a dinner plate or smaller.* Larger predatory fish tend to have higher concentrations of mercury and PCBs because more polluted water has circulated through their gills, and they have ingested more contaminated fish. So choose smaller fish: They'll have spent less time in polluted waters and should have lower concentrations of mercury and PCBs

that farmed salmon have sixteen times more PCBs than wild salmon.

On pages 174–175, you'll find a list of fish with the highest and lowest mercury levels, and you can download an app, such as the one created by the Environmental Defense Fund, to keep the list with you at all times.

In light of mercury and PCB contamination, the current government recommendations suggest limiting fish intake to no more than two meals per week.

OVERFISHING

Overfishing occurs when more fish are caught than the population is able to replenish through natural methods of reproduction and can lead to extinction. This is a real threat to a number of species, including Atlantic halibut and bluefin tuna.

Overfishing does more than just wipe out an entire species. When large predatory fish, such as tuna, are overfished, the natural ecosystem is also disrupted, resulting in larger populations of smaller fish, such as sardines and anchovies. This, in turn, can lead to increased algae growth and may damage coral reef health.

SEAFOOD

Overfishing also results in the needless deaths of billions of fish, turtles, and crustaceans that aren't used as food but get caught in the net accidentally. This is called bycatch, and it further disrupts the ecosystem. It's a serious threat to the stability and well-being of our oceans.

Seafood Shopping & Storage Tips

- As with meat and poultry, pick up fish last when you're at the grocery store so it won't become warm in your shopping cart.

- If it takes you more than thirty minutes to travel home, place the fish in a cooler with ice. Refrigerate or freeze immediately when you get home.

- Place fish on the refrigerator's bottom shelf in a closed plastic bag to prevent any liquid from leaking onto other foods.

- Cook within one to two days or freeze. Fatty fish such as salmon can be frozen for two to three months, while lean fish will last up to six months.

How to Select Seafood

Here are the best ways to choose seafood varies by species. The following tips will help you get the freshest seafood every time.

1. Choose wild and line or pole-caught fish, which tend to be higher in nutrients and lower in chemicals that are best avoided, such as PCBs and mercury. The standards for organic fish are not well defined, so these are better options.

2. Choose fish the size of a dinner plate or smaller to limit mercury intake.

3. Frozen fish are okay—and may even be better! More than 70 percent of "fresh" fish has been frozen at some point, according to the National Fisheries Institute, including 100 percent of all wild fish. So save money and buy it frozen instead of purchasing defrosted fish at the fish market.

CLAMS, OYSTERS & MUSSELS

- Do the tap test: Live clams, oysters, and mussels will naturally gape, but will close tightly when tapped. If it doesn't close, don't buy it.

- Avoid shellfish with cracked or broken shells.

- Freshly shucked oysters will be surrounded by a slightly milky or light gray liquid.

CRABS & LOBSTER

Look for leg movement: Crabs and lobsters spoil rapidly after death, so they should only be selected, purchased, and cooked if alive.

FRESH FISH

- Fish should smell fresh and salty, like the ocean—not strong and "fishy."

- If the head is still on, the eyes should be bright, shiny, clear, and slightly bulging. Cloudy or sunken eyes indicate the fish is not fresh.

- Look for firm, shiny flesh that bounces back when pressed.

- The freshest fish have bright, metallic skin. Avoid any that are patchy or dull.

- The gills should be bright red. As a fish ages, the gills will turn brown. Slimy gills are a sure sign it's past its prime.

- Fillets of fish should be moist with no discoloration. They should be bright and firm, not soft or dull.

❗ Expert Tip

Suggested Serving Size Guidelines for Seafood	
Serving size:	3 to 4 ounces (85 to 115 g), about the size of an iPhone 6
Servings per day:	None to one
Frequency per week:	Up to two meals per week

FROZEN SEAFOOD

- Frozen seafood is a good choice. You save money with frozen seafood and still get all the nutrition.

- Don't buy packages with signs of frost or ice crystals, which may mean it has been stored for a long time or has been thawed and refrozen. Frozen seafood can spoil if it thaws during transport or if it's left at warm temperatures for too long.

SHRIMP

- Shrimp should be translucent and shiny, smell fresh, and feel firm.

CHAPTER 10

EGGS

Whether scrambled, hardboiled, or folded into an omelet, eggs are a breakfast staple. This versatile food is a good source of B vitamins, including vitamin B_{12}, as well as a variety of minerals, such as selenium, zinc, iron, and phosphorus.

You can give your breakfast a healthy boost by taking a hint from Dr. Seuss: Make "green eggs" by stuffing or scrambling your eggs with dark leafy greens, such as spinach, chard, or broccoli. It's an easy and delicious way to sneak in some veggies, bringing you that much closer to your daily requirements. Onions, garlic, and fresh herbs go well with eggs, too.

When purchasing eggs, don't fear the dizzying number of terms on the carton: "cage free," "pasture raised," and "omega-3 enriched," to name a few. This chapter explains them all! Like all animal products, it's important to be selective and look for quality.

Egg Buzzwords

Because there are so many egg-related buzzwords, they're divided here into **living standards** and **food standards** because the living standard terms don't give an indication of feed and vice versa. Aside for the term "organic," the living standards terms are not USDA-regulated, so they can be used loosely.

When purchasing eggs, look for certifications such as "Animal Welfare Approved" or "Certified Humane" to ensure third-party verification of the highest standards.

Also, to understand these terms better, you need to know about the standard conditions in which egg-laying hens are raised. Conventional eggs come from factory farms where the hens live in small battery cages—about the size of a sheet of paper—without much room to move or perform natural behaviors, like walking or spreading their wings.

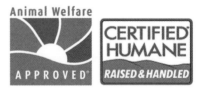

The following buzzwords pertain to living standards.

CAGE FREE
"Cage free" signifies the animals are not kept in tiny battery cages, but it does not mean they live outside, nor does it provide an indication of their diet.

FREE RANGE/FREE ROAMING
Typically, free-range hens are cage free inside barns and have some degree of outdoor access, but the amount of time spent outdoors is not defined and could be minimal. (These are a better choice.)

PASTURE RAISED

Typically, pasture-raised hens are allowed outdoors on a spacious pasture during the day and taken inside at night. This allows them to forage for food on the pasture, which is their natural habit. Studies show that eggs from pasture-raised chickens have twice the amount of vitamin E and nearly three times the amount of omega-3 than eggs from caged hens due to their more natural diet. Note this is not currently a USDA-regulated term, so it may be used loosely by farmers.

These buzzwords pertain to food standards.

OMEGA-3 ENRICHED

Omega-3 enriched eggs come from hens fed a diet rich in omega-3s, which could come from flaxseed, fish oil, or algae. A regular egg typically has about fifty milligrams of omega-3s, and an egg from a hen with an enriched diet can have between three to five times that amount. Pasture-raised eggs also, generally, have twice the amount of omega-3s as a standard egg—simply because the hen had a naturally foraged diet.

VEGETARIAN FED

Vegetarian-fed hens eat a diet containing no animal products. This is not necessarily a good thing, as hens are not naturally vegetarians, and this means they were not able to forage for their natural diet of worms and bugs.

This buzzword pertains to both living and food standards.

ORGANIC

Certified organic eggs come from hens that do not live in battery cages and do have outdoor access, although the amount of time they spend outside isn't defined. The hens must be fed organic feed free from antibiotics,

◎ **Myth Alert!**

Myth: Egg whites are healthier than whole eggs.

Fact: Most of the nutrition derived from eggs is found in the yolk, so throwing it out is a waste. The trend for egg whites began over concerns regarding cholesterol, but we now know that dietary cholesterol is not the true culprit behind heart disease. Plus, egg whites sold in cartons are derived using chemical extraction methods and are less than ideal. If you need egg whites for a specific recipe, separate them yourself and be sure to reserve the yolk for another use.

pesticides, animal byproducts, and GMOs. This is the golden standard, or buzzword, you should look for.

Finding & Selecting High-Quality Eggs

When selecting eggs, consider the following:

- Choose organic.

- Choose pasture-raised or free-range eggs. Pasture-raised is ideal because the hen's lifestyle will be most natural—and, therefore, healthiest. If you can't find pasture-raised, opt for free-range.

The best sources of high-quality eggs include the following:

- Farmers' markets
- Health food stores
- Direct from small, local farms

    Or, check out www.eatwild.com/products/index.html to find local producers near you.

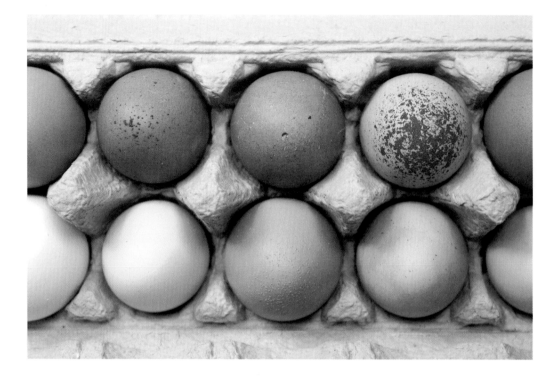

Egg Colors

An egg's color is determined by the breed of hen that lays it. While you'll probably find only white and brown eggs in the grocery store, you may see eggs in a variety of colors ranging from rose to blue to green to black at a farmers' market. And, in case you're wondering, brown eggs are not any more nutritious or natural than white ones: They're simply laid by a different breed of hen!

Benefits of Eggs

There is no need to fear the cholesterol in eggs, as science now shows us that eating eggs in moderation does not contribute to increased risk of heart disease or stroke. In fact, whole eggs offer a number of health benefits.

VITAMIN B$_{12}$

Eggs contain vitamin B$_{12}$, an essential nutrient that supports the nervous system and new red blood cell formation. A deficiency in B$_{12}$ can lead to anemia, memory loss, and even dementia.

COMPLETE PROTEIN

Eggs are a complete source of protein because they contain all the essential amino acids our bodies need.

CHOLINE

Eggs are the richest source of choline, a mineral necessary for cognitive and healthy organ function, particularly in older adults. It's also crucial for pregnant and breast-feeding women, as a deficiency could lead to impaired fetal brain and memory development.

Concerns About Eggs

Though the most common fear surrounding eggs—too much dietary cholesterol can lead to cardiac issues—is based on outdated science and no longer considered an issue, there are other, more pressing concerns that you should be aware of when purchasing and consuming eggs.

SALMONELLA

Salmonella is a bacteria that can cause diarrhea, fever, and abdominal cramps, which can last up to a week. It can be fatal in children, the elderly, and those with weakened immune systems. Both the exterior and interior of an egg may contain salmonella. Because of the filthy conditions in conventional factory farms, it's quite easy for it to be spread. A 2010 study published in *Veterinary Record* found that eggs from hens confined to cages were nearly eight times more likely to contain salmonella than eggs from non-caged hens. To limit risk of salmonella exposure, choose free-range or pastured eggs and cook them thoroughly.

ANTIBIOTICS

Conventional hens are given antibiotics to make them grow faster and prevent illness in the close quarters and filthy conditions in which they live. Antibiotics may then end up in your eggs, where they've been linked to antibiotic resistance and even obesity.

❗ Expert Tip

Suggested Serving Size Guidelines for Eggs	
Serving Size	Two eggs
Servings per day	One, up to three to four times a week

Note: *The Dietary Guidelines for Americans* doesn't provide a specific serving size or frequency for eating eggs, noting that dietary cholesterol is no longer believed to be a cause for concern. The United Kingdom has no recommended limit when eggs are included as part of an overall healthy and balanced diet.

In terms of research, at least two studies have indicated that moderate egg consumption—on average one whole egg a day, or up to seven eggs per week—doesn't have adverse cardiac effects in healthy people. (Although it was linked with a higher risk of cardiovascular disease in diabetics.) There hasn't been much research on consumption of more than two eggs a day. However, when relying on eggs as the protein source for a meal, it's more likely that two to three eggs are used, hence the larger serving size recommended here.

EGGS

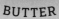
BUTTER

CHEDDAR

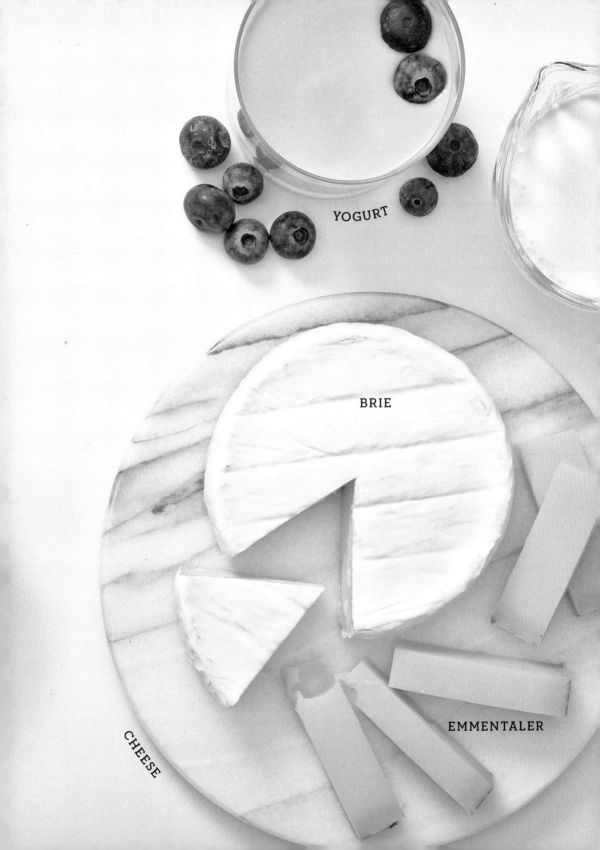

YOGURT

BRIE

CHEESE

EMMENTALER

CHAPTER 11

DAIRY

Dairy is ingrained in many Western cultures. We pour milk on our breakfast cereal and in our coffee. We layer cheese on sandwiches and devour cheese-laden pizza. The U.S. government subsidizes the milk served with school lunches.

Our love affair with dairy is real, but waning. In recent years, nondairy alternatives, such as almond milk, cashew cheese, and coconut ice cream, have enjoyed surges in popularity. It's likely this switch to plant-based alternatives is due to a number of reasons. For one thing, some people find dairy hard to digest or notice that it contributes to other health concerns, such as acne, inflammation, or chronic mucus. Also, its position as the go-to drink for strong bones has been challenged, as research and population studies suggest otherwise. And plant-based alternatives offer similar flavors and textures—without the same health concerns.

In short, it turns out dairy products aren't the health foods they were once cracked up to be. Paradoxically, milk has even been found to weaken bones when intake is high. High intake has been linked to an increased risk of prostate, and probably ovarian, cancer. Whether you choose to consume dairy is up to you, and this chapter helps you make an informed decision.

Milk Buzzwords

There are a number of types of milk and ways of raising dairy cows. The terms following will help you understand what you're buying in the dairy aisle.

WHOLE MILK

Whole milk is the traditional full-fat form of milk. It's creamier, more satisfying, and more nutritious than lower-fat versions.

LOW-FAT MILK/TWO-PERCENT MILK/ ONE-PERCENT MILK

Two-percent milk is created when some fat is removed from whole milk, creating a lower-calorie—yet also less nutritious—milk. One-percent contains even less fat, calories, and nutrients. Both are usually fortified with vitamins A and D to make up for the vitamin loss during processing.

SKIM MILK/FAT-FREE MILK

Skim or fat-free milk contains 0 to 0.5 percent fat. Skim milk is always fortified with vitamins A and D because, even though whole milk contains considerable amounts of both, they're removed with the cream during processing because they're fat-soluble. And too much synthetic vitamin A can have negative health consequences. When compared with regular milk, skim milk has been associated with a higher risk of developing acne and excess weight. Overall, this may be the least healthy type of milk.

HOMOGENIZED

Homogenization is a mechanical process that occurs after pasteurization, in which the fat molecules in milk are broken down so they resist separation, resulting in a smoother consistency and taste. (Naturally, the fat molecules would rise to the top, creating a thick layer of cream.) In general, all milk sold at grocery stores is homogenized.

PASTEURIZED

Milk is pasteurized to kill any harmful bacteria and ensure safety. It extends milk's shelf life to two to three weeks. A common method of pasteurization is to heat milk to a high temperature (162°F, or 72°C) for fifteen seconds and then rapidly cool it. Generally, all milk sold in grocery stores is pasteurized.

ORGANIC

Organic milk comes from cows fed an organic diet—free of pesticides and GMOs. These animals are not given synthetic hormones or antibiotics and should have continuous access to pasture.

GRASS FED

Milk from grass-fed cows contains higher amounts of essential omega-3 fatty acids and generally comes from healthier cows as they enjoy their natural diet.

HORMONE FREE

Hormone-free milk is from cows not given synthetic hormones, which they often receive to increase milk production. Aside from the fact that they may end up in your milk, hormones

FACT **What's Causing Your Dairy Sensitivity?**

One of these factors may be at the root of your dairy sensitivity:

- **Lactose intolerance:** This is the body's inability to digest lactose, a sugar in milk, due to the body's lack of lactase, a digestive enzyme. With lactose intolerance, digestive upset—including bloating, gas, and diarrhea—typically ensues after consuming dairy.

- **Milk allergy:** Milk allergies occur when the immune system identifies milk proteins, most commonly alpha s1 casein, as invaders that must be attacked. Symptoms include wheezing, vomiting, hives, runny nose, itchy skin, and digestive problems. Milk allergies are among the most common food allergies, particularly in children.

make the cows more susceptible to contracting mastitis, an udder infection caused by overpumping—which, inevitably, leads to the use of even more antibiotics. This is why hormone-free and organic milk are better choices.

GOAT'S MILK/SHEEP'S MILK

Goat's and sheep's milk contain less lactose than cow's milk as well as less alpha s1 casein protein, which is what causes milk allergies in some people (the body's immune system sees it as an invader and fights it off similar to the way it would a cold or flu virus). While people with lactose intolerance or milk allergies may find it easier to digest, the same general concerns regarding cow's milk hold true for goat's and sheep's milk. A plant-based alternative may be a better option.

Cheese, Yogurt & Ice Cream Buzzwords

As with milk, learning the meaning behind these common food terms helps you make the best choices at the store.

LOW FAT

In low-fat dairy products, some of the fat has been removed. This tends to make foods such as yogurt and cheese unpalatable, so refined sugar or refined salt is often added to improve taste. This makes such products less healthy and less satisfying. Whole-fat products are a better choice.

NO-FAT/FAT-FREE

At least 99.5 percent of the fat has been removed from these dairy products. To make up for the lack of flavor, copious amounts of refined sugar or refined salt are often added. These additives make no-fat and fat-free products the least healthy type of dairy products overall.

Concerns About Dairy

You may notice that I haven't preceded the concerns with the usual benefits. That's because, in my opinion, the concerns surrounding dairy outweigh its possible benefits. Understanding those concerns can help you decide how much, if any, dairy to include in your diet.

OSTEOPOROSIS

You may have grown up with the *Got Milk?* ads, which claimed that milk "does a body good" and that it creates strong bones through its calcium content. But, as it turns out, the countries with the highest dairy consumption also have the highest osteoporosis rates, including the United States, the United Kingdom, Finland, and Sweden. On the other hand, bone fractures and osteoporosis are

❗ Expert Tip

Build Strong Bones

Move beyond the dairy aisle to support strong bones and reduce your risk of osteoporosis with these tips:

- Include dark leafy greens in your diet every day. They supply calcium, magnesium, and vitamin K, all of which support healthy bones.

- Soak up some vitamin D. Dubbed the "sunshine vitamin," vitamin D is essential for strong and healthy bones. Your body produces it naturally when your skin is exposed to the sun—although it's also available in supplement form.

- Exercise regularly—every day. Weight-bearing exercise, such as walking, jogging, stair climbing, and weight training, are crucial to building strong bones.

- Avoid excessive preformed vitamin A, or retinol, which is found in meat, poultry, fish, and dairy products, plus fortified foods and supplements. It has been associated with decreased bone density and increased risk of osteoporosis. This does not apply to vitamin A from plant-based foods, so rely on vegetables for your vitamin A and avoid excessive animal product consumption.

minimal in countries where dairy consumption is low, such as India, Japan, and Peru.

Some researchers believe the culprit behind this apparent paradox is the very nature of dairy itself. Although it's high in calcium, it's also high in retinol (vitamin A) and protein, both of which can contribute to the leaching of calcium and other minerals from the bones.

The truth is, we don't necessarily need dairy in our diet. The Harvard School of Public Health doesn't even include it on its *Healthy Eating Plate*. It acknowledges there are better sources of calcium available, such as dark leafy greens and beans, and recommend limiting all forms of dairy—including milk, cheese, ice cream, milk, etc.—to a maximum of one to two daily servings.

LACTOSE INTOLERANCE
Virtually all infants and young children have lactase (an enzyme that helps the body digest lactose), and scientists once believed all adults have it, too. However, in the 1960s scientists began to test this hypothesis and the results proved otherwise. Studies suggested that as many as 90 percent of Asian Americans, 70 percent of African Americans, and 53 percent of Mexican Americans do not have lactase and so are unable to digest milk. People of Jewish, Italian, and Greek heritage may also experience a substantial decrease in lactase as they age.

In 1988, research published in the *American Journal of Clinical Nutrition* reported: "It rapidly became apparent that this pattern was the genetic norm, and that lactase activity was sustained only in a majority of adults whose origins were in Northern Europe or some Mediterranean populations." According to the Physicians Committee for Responsible Medicine, it's estimated that as much as 75 percent of the world's population loses its lactase enzymes after weaning.

So, while some people can digest dairy as adults, others cannot. If you have trouble digesting dairy and experience digestive distress or other side effects as a result of eating it, consider avoiding it.

PROSTATE & OVARIAN CANCER RISKS
Studies show that dairy consumption may be linked to an increased risk of both prostate and ovarian cancers. Multiple cohort studies have linked milk and prostate cancer as early as the 1970s. In 2000 Harvard published a study that followed more than twenty thousand men for eleven years and found that two and a half servings of dairy per day increased the risk of prostate cancer by 34 percent, compared to less than one-half serving daily.

Much more research on the connection between dairy and ovarian cancer is necessary, but there is some evidence that would suggest a possible link. A recent large analysis of twelve prospective cohort studies that included more than 500,000 women found those with the highest lactose intakes had a modestly higher risk of ovarian cancer compared to those with the lowest lactose intakes. The high lactose amount was the equivalent of three cups (700 ml) of milk per day, which is the recommended daily value proposed by the USDA.

THE RAW MILK DEBATE
There is a growing movement in support of raw milk, which is milk that has not been pasteurized or homogenized. Supporters believe it not only tastes better, but is healthier and more nutritious than the processed stuff found on grocery store shelves. However, in the United States, the CDC and FDA are very much opposed to it, citing its increased risk for pathogen contamination, such as salmonella, E.coli, and *Listeria*. In fact, bacterial contamination of milk was the very reason pasteurization was developed. The retail sale of raw milk is currently legal in only ten states and illegal in seven. Laws for the remaining states are somewhere in between.

Globally, raw milk for human consumption is banned completely in Australia and Scotland (where multiple people died from its consumption in 1983). In Germany and England, it is allowed but restricted. A farmer is able to sell his raw milk direct to a consumer, but it must come with a health-warning label. In France, raw milk sales are allowed, and you can even buy it out of vending machines. Plus, as much as 18 percent of French cheese is made the traditional way—with raw milk. Even where allowed, raw products still only make up a small percentage of the overall milk production and consumption.

Regardless of availability, studies in favor of raw milk, so far, have been small and inconclusive; the risk of bacterial contamination is higher, and there are a number of larger studies linking dairy consumption to decreased bone density and osteoporosis and even certain cancers. So, raw milk may taste better, but may not be worth the risk.

BUTTER IS NOT BACK

In March 2014, an article stating that eating less saturated fat *did not* lower the risk of heart disease—as was thought to be the case at the time—appeared in the *Annals of Internal Medicine*. The foodie community took this as a green light to bring butter back in full force. But the subsequent media headlines, which suggested we'd been unnecessarily avoiding butter (and burgers) for all those years, were misguided. Yes, it's true that the amount of saturated fat in a food may not have the same implications we once thought it did, but it's imperative that we look at the whole food, not just its macronutrient parts.

The fact remains that other foods lead to healthier outcomes, in comparison with butter. According to Walter Willet, M.D., Dr.P.H., chair of the nutrition department at Harvard School of Public Health, "Butter is not back. Long-term health will be better with olive oil and other oils (sorry Julia [Child])." As for the butter-in-coffee trend? There is no scientific evidence to support the idea that adding butter to coffee boosts energy or helps with weight loss. Because fat does slow digestion, it may slow the absorption of caffeine into the bloodstream, which could result in more

sustained energy levels, instead of the quick high and low you typically get from caffeine on its own.

After assessing the health concerns associated with dairy, if you choose to consume it, there are helpful guidelines for doing so. And if you're ready to ditch dairy, an extensive list of nondairy alternatives can be found in chapter 17.

Types of Dairy

Dairy comes in many forms, from savory to sweet. Here are the best practices for choosing each.

BUTTER/MARGARINE

Butter is a concentrated source of dairy fat and is best replaced with healthy oils, according to Walter Willet. Try replacing butter with olive, avocado, or coconut oil.

Avoid margarine completely as consumption has been shown to increase heart attack risk by 53 percent.

Avoid dairy-free or fake butters which are typically made from inferior oils.

CHEESE

Cheese is a high-calorie product that's about 70 percent fat and loaded with salt, a combo that makes it a hard habit to kick. Worse, it can be constipating and cause digestive discomfort, including gas and bloating. That said, if you're going to eat it, at least eat the real thing.

Real cheese is made by heating milk, stirring in enzymes and cultures, separating the curds from the whey, adding salt, and, finally, shaping the curds into a block or wheel to age. This means anything neon-orange in color or wrapped in plastic is, typically, not real cheese. Look closely at the package, and you'll see it's called something like "pasteurized process cheese," "pasteurized process cheese product," or "pasteurized process cheese food."

"Cheese food" is a blend of premade cheeses that are reheated, pasteurized, and mixed with an emulsifier—and possibly other ingredients—to manipulate texture, taste, and mouthfeel. Light cheeses can have up to twenty ingredients added to make them *semi*-palatable. Because of this, you may want to avoid processed cheese foods, including string cheese, American cheese, and imitation cheese shreds. Instead, choose high-quality, traditionally made, or European-style cheeses.

CREAM

Cream is the milk fat skimmed off two-percent, one-percent, and skim milk. Heavy cream or heavy whipping cream is about 36 percent fat, while whipping cream is about 30 percent fat. The more fat it contains, the more the cream whips. A delicious nondairy alternative to cream can be made from coconut milk or coconut butter.

HALF-AND-HALF

Half-and-half is a blend of equal parts whole milk and cream and is typically used in coffee. Nonfat half-and-half is a blend of nonfat milk

with corn syrup and thickeners, making it a doubly bad choice, in my opinion.

ICE CREAM

It's pretty obvious that ice cream isn't a health food, but there are, indeed, healthier alternatives to it (and by now you can probably guess I'm not talking about low-fat or fat-free ice creams!). Coconut and nut-based, nondairy ice creams offer a smiliar texture and flavor without the concerns associated with dairy.

MILK

Milk needs no introduction (although I bet you're already thinking differently about it!). If you do decide to drink milk, organic whole milk, ideally from a local farm, is best. If you're reassessing your milk consumption, there are a number of alternative, dairy-free milks on the market. Just watch out for strange additives. For tips on choosing the best nondairy milks, see chapter 17.

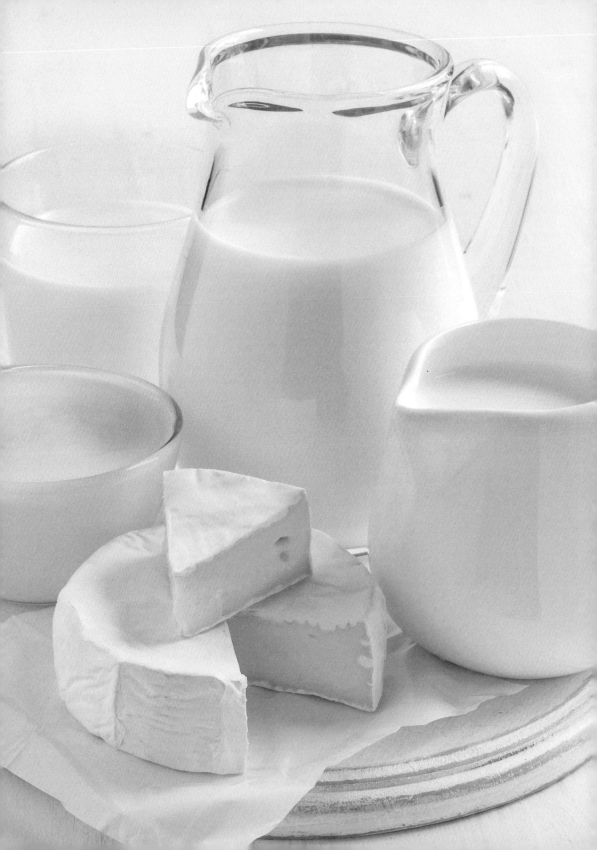

YOGURT

Of all the forms of dairy, yogurt tends to be the easiest to digest because it's fermented and should contain probiotics. To make sure you actually get the probiotics, check that the label says "contains" live active cultures, not simply "made with" live active cultures. Greek yogurt may be better, as it's lower in sugar. There are a number of great coconut yogurt alternatives, too.

KEFIR

Kefir is a cultured probiotic drink, similar to yogurt but thinner in consistency. The main difference is the type of bacterial cultures used. Kefir typically contains a larger range of bacteria and, unlike yogurt, also contains yeast. The bacteria in kefir are capable of colonizing the intestinal tract, while those in yogurt simply provide food for the bacteria already there and simply pass through without taking up residence.

Selecting Milk, Cheese, Yogurt & Kefir

- Choose organic.

- Choose whole or full-fat versions. Full-fat cheese is less processed and more satisfying.

- Avoid "processed cheese foods." Avoid anything called "pasteurized process cheese," "pasteurized process cheese product," or "pasteurized process cheese food," including American cheese, string cheese, and imitation cheese shreds.

! Expert Tip

Suggested Serving Size Guidelines for Dairy	
Serving size	One cup of milk (235 ml) or yogurt (230 g); 1.5 ounces (42 g) natural cheese
Servings per day	Up to two

- Avoid flavored milks and yogurts. Products such as chocolate milk and strawberry yogurt tend to contain a lot of added sugar, which should be avoided. Instead, add your own fresh fruit toppings to yogurt or make your own chocolate milk with cocoa powder and, perhaps, a pinch of coconut sugar or maple syrup.

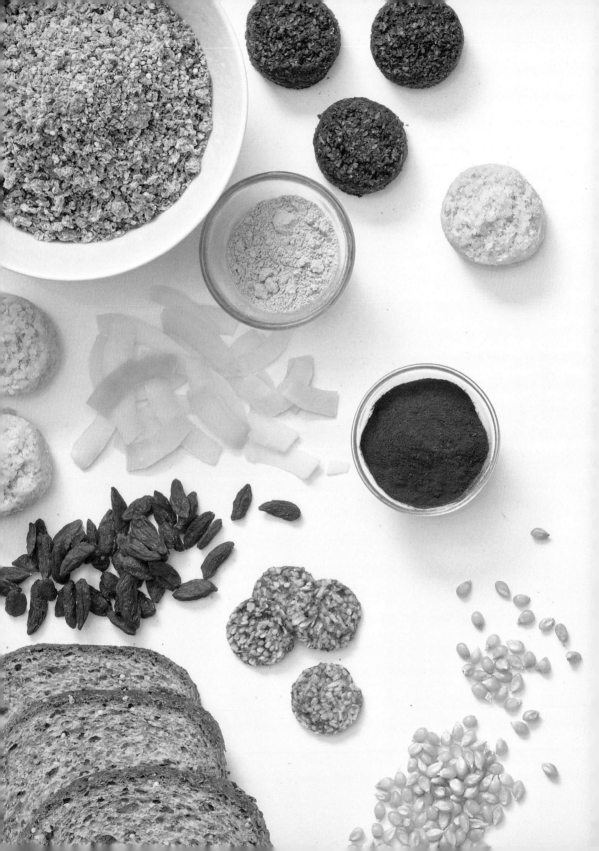

PART IV

PACKAGED FOODS

Ditch the Junk & Make Better Choices. If you are what you eat, do you really want to eat azodicarbonamide, antifreeze, or cow poop extract?

Nope, I didn't think so. But the packaged food aisles have turned into something of a minefield. You never know what's really lurking inside each pretty package until you read the ingredients list—and even that may require a dictionary, three apps, and a food scientist to decipher. Though whole foods are better for you, nothing beats the convenience of preprepared and packaged foods, especially in our hectic, busy lives. Luckily, not all packaged foods are junk.

You no longer have to choose between convenience and health. This section teaches you how to evaluate any packaged food so you can choose the healthiest option. It may take a little sleuthing to find the right brands and products, but they're out there, and this section helps you find them. (For even more guidance, plus brand recommendations, head to www.mariamarlowe.com/real-food-guide.)

CHAPTER 12

HOW TO CHOOSE PACKAGED FOODS

It's true. The closer we come to eating real, whole foods, the better. But, sometimes, modern life calls for packaged foods, which are convenient and fast. Unfortunately, most packaged foods are loaded with salt, sugar, chemicals, and unhealthy fats. They're typically high in calories yet devoid of nutrients, making them the perfect recipe for poor health, weight gain, and chronic disease.

Luckily not all packaged foods are created equal. In this chapter, you'll learn to ascertain the true health value of any packaged product, so you'll be able to choose the healthiest ones—every time.

We'll start with a breakdown of the many buzzwords you're likely to see on the front of food packages, so you know how to distinguish fluff from fact.

You'll also learn exactly what those items on the Nutrition Facts Panel mean and why, contrary to popular belief, the Nutrition Facts Panel is not the best indicator of the health value of a product.

Next, you'll learn how to decipher the ingredients list and discover why it's the most significant aspect of any food package.

Finally, we end with a discussion of the things you may want to avoid, including some of the most controversial food additives, genetically modified organisms (GMOs), and canned foods.

Packaged Foods Buzzwords

Packaged foods have become billboards for food and health buzzwords, sporting lists of their attributes—such as "natural," "organic," and "gluten-free." Some of the terms used to describe food have real meaning, while others are essentially fluffy marketing terms used to coax consumers into purchasing a product that's probably less healthy than it seems.

As you read this list, note that none of the terms necessarily signifies the health quality of a food product. For example, you can now find prepackaged organic cookies, but I wouldn't be that keen on swapping them for an organic apple. The terms simply tell you what the item *does* or *does not* contain. The best way to ascertain the health value of a packaged product is to read the ingredients list, discussed on page 205.

FAIR TRADE

The fair trade stamp certifies that the farmers and workers who made the product were fairly compensated. It may not improve your health, but it'll surely improve the lives of the people who grew your food!

GENERALLY RECOGNIZED AS SAFE (GRAS)

GRAS is not a term you'll see on the front of a package, but you'll come across it in the discussion of ingredients in packaged foods. It's an FDA designation indicating that a chemical or substance is considered safe by the FDA and so is allowed to be used as a food additive.

GLUTEN FREE

Gluten-free foods do not contain the protein gluten or grains that contain gluten, such as wheat, barley, rye, spelt, kamut, farro, durum, bulgur, or semolina. Gluten-free products are typically made from the flours of rice, beans, nuts, or seeds, but are not necessarily healthy (although they could be!). While the ingredients of a gluten-free product may not contain gluten, if it's made in a facility that processes gluten-containing products, there is a chance that it may be cross-contaminated with gluten.

CERTIFIED GLUTEN-FREE

 Certified gluten-free foods are made in a dedicated gluten-free facility, eliminating the chance for any cross-contamination. If you have a serious gluten allergy or suffer from celiac disease, always look for a certified gluten-free seal.

LOCAL

Local foods are grown or raised within a small geographic radius, typically within 50 to 150 miles (80 to 241 km) of wherever you're purchasing it. Local packaged foods help protect the environment by reducing carbon dioxide emissions due to shipping, and they also strengthen your local economy.

ORGANIC

 Packaged foods with organic ingredients are held to the same strict standards as fresh foods. They have been produced *without* the use of pesticides or GMOs—or antibiotics and growth hormones, for animal ingredients.

Packaged foods that sport the green and white USDA organic seal are made with at least 95 percent organic ingredients. If you see "made with organic ingredients" on the box, it indicates the product contains at least 70 percent organic ingredients. Turn over the box and read the ingredients list to see just which ingredients are organic.

While organic foods are preferable to conventional ones, don't assume that any organic packaged food is automatically healthy. Organic cookies, for example, may be made with organic ingredients, but they generally contain just as much sugar, as many calories, and as many refined ingredients as their conventional counterparts.

NATURAL

The word "natural" is not defined or regulated by the FDA, so it may not mean much on a food package. It can be found on products that don't contain all-natural ingredients. If you see this term on packaged goods, be suspicious: More often than not, unscrupulous companies use the term to make you think you're getting a healthier product than you actually are.

NON-GMO

 Non-GMO foods do not contain genetically modified organisms. GMOs are discussed in greater detail later in this chapter (see page 212), but, in short, GMO crops are suspected to pose harm to humans and the environment and are banned or labeled in many countries. To avoid GMOs, look for the Non-GMO Project seal or the USDA Organic seal on any foods that contain *corn, soy, canola, beet sugar,* or *sugar*, the most common genetically modified crops found in packaged foods.

Be wary of products that say they are non-GMO but do not contain this seal. (If a packaged food doesn't contain one of these ingredients, then the seal is not as important, as most other ingredients are non-GMO by default.) Without third-party verification, it's impossible to know whether the products are truly non-GMO without sending them to a lab—and there have been instances in which manufacturers have claimed that a product was non-GMO when it wasn't.

PALEO

Paleo is a popular style of eating based on the idea that we should only eat what our ancestors ate. It includes fruit, vegetables, lean meats, seafood, nuts, seeds, and healthy fats. It does not include dairy, grains, processed foods, sugar, legumes, starch, or alcohol.

Although the basis for the diet is controversial (see page 122), the main tenet—eat whole foods of the highest quality and avoid sugar and processed foods—is spot-on. Paradoxically, though, even though whole foods form the basis of Paleo, people still love convenience, so you'll now see packaged Paleo products on the market—from granola

to pizza crusts. Products that truly stick to the Paleo guidelines will typically be healthy choices as they won't contain refined sugars or chemical fillers.

RAW

The term "raw" refers to any food item that has not been cooked at a temperature higher than 118°F (47.8°C). It's either unprocessed or minimally processed. You'll find it most often on vegan snacks and desserts, such as crackers made from seeds, dehydrated vegetable chips, or pies made from fruits and nuts. Raw food desserts, made with whole ingredients, are usually a better choice than traditional cookies and cakes.

PLANT BASED

Plant-based foods are those that come entirely from plant sources: vegetables, fruit, seeds, nuts, grains, or legumes. A plant-based diet is one in which the majority or entirety of one's diet consists of plant-based foods.

VEGAN

Vegan foods do not contain any animal products, such as meat, dairy, eggs, or honey. "Vegan" does not necessarily mean "healthy," and these products can still contain unhealthy ingredients, such as sugar or refined flours.

VEGETARIAN

Vegetarian foods do not contain meat or fish, but may contain dairy, eggs, or honey. They can still contain unhealthy ingredients, such as sugar or refined flours, so be aware that "vegetarian" isn't always synonymous with "healthy."

WHOLE FOOD

Not to be confused with the grocery store called Whole Foods Market, a whole food is simply a food in its natural, unprocessed form, such as fresh fruit, vegetables, raw nuts and seeds, grains, legumes, and unprocessed meat.

How to Read a Food Label

Between twenty-six-letter ingredients and bullet-point lists of buzzwords on food packages, you may feel in need of a crash course in "Food as a Second Language." There is an overwhelming amount of packaged-food products in grocery stores. And as we're usually rushing to get in and out of the store quickly, we tend to operate on autopilot: We may glance at the front of a box, maybe scan the Nutrition Facts panel to check the calorie count, and throw it into our basket without a second thought. This way of shopping, however, is not the most health supportive.

Contrary to common belief, the best way to ascertain the health value of a product is to *read the ingredients list*, not the Nutrition Facts panel. Simply looking at a food product's macronutrients can be misleading, and the habit is based on outdated science and assumptions. More and more research has shown that the quality of a calorie—meaning its source—is a better indicator of its effect on the body than the quantity of calories a food contains. Old habits die hard, though, so we'll first take a look at the Nutrition Facts panel and what it means before taking a closer look at the ingredients list.

NUTRITION FACTS PANEL

Number of calories and grams of fat alone do not give you an accurate indicator of the healthiness of a product. ▶

Nutrition Facts
Serving Size 13 crackers (30g)
Servings Per Container about 6

Amount Per Serving

Calories 140	Calories From Fat 45

	% Daily Value*
Total Fat 5g	8%
Saturated Fat** 0.5g	3%
Polyunsaturated Fat 2.5g	
Monounsaturated Fat 1.5g	
Trans Fat 0g	
Cholesterol 0mg	0%
Sodium 190mg	8%
Total Carbs 21g	7%
Dietary Fiber 3g	12%
Sugars 0g	
Proteins 3g	20%

Vitamin A **0%**	•	Vitamin C **0%**	
Calcium **15%**	•	Iron **1%**	

*Percent Daily Values are based on a 2,000 calorie diet.

◀ Out of every item listed on the panel, sugar is probably the one you should be most concerned with.

Made with unique & nutritious ingredients:

Ingredients: Organic whole grain brown rice, organic whole grain quinoa, organic brown flax seeds, organic brown sesame seeds, filtered water, organic minced dried onions, sea salt, organic wheat free tamari (water, whole organic soybeans, salt, organic alcohol or organic vinegar).

Contains: Soy

This is the most important part of any packaged food: **INGREDIENTS.** ▶

NEW NUTRITION FACTS PANEL
(Coming 2018)

At the time of writing, the Nutrition Facts panel—as we know it—was under scrutiny. By May 2016, the FDA announced that a new Nutrition Facts panel is to be implemented on July 26, 2018.

This change is the result of an effort to reflect new scientific information, including the link between diet and chronic diseases such as obesity and heart disease. While it's a definite improvement over the original—especially because it will require more realistic serving sizes and will differentiate between the amount of added sugar versus natural sugar in a product—you still should not rely upon it alone to ascertain a product's healthiness.

So what's different?

Serving size—larger, bolder type. The serving size is much more prominent.

Breaks out added sugars and includes percentage of daily value (DV). *This is significant* because naturally occurring sugar is different than added refined sugar. The label

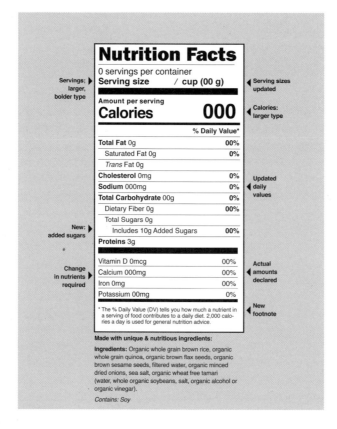

Source: www.fda.gov/Food/GuidanceRegulation/
GuidanceDocumentsRegulatoryInformation/LabelingNutrition/ucm385663.htm

will include the amount both in grams and as a percentage of DV, which may help curb excessive sugar consumption. For example, a twenty-ounce (570 ml) bottle of soda will say it contains 130 percent DV for added sugar, which may deter people from buying it and may even cause manufacturers to reformulate it so it contains less sugar.

Removal of "Calories from Fat." This is being removed because research shows that the type of fat consumed is more import-ant than the amount of fat. (See "Partially Hydrogenated Oils/Trans Fat" on page 209 for more information.)

Change in nutrients required. Vitamins A and C no longer have to be listed on the label, while vitamin D and potassium do. This is because vitamin A and C deficiencies are rare, while CDC surveys suggest Americans don't always get enough vitamin D and potassium. Lack of both of these vitamins is associated with chronic disease.

Serving sizes updated. Serving sizes are being updated to better reflect what a person actually eats in one sitting. For example, one large cookie will comprise one serving instead of two and both a twelve-ounce (355 ml) and a twenty-ounce (570 ml) soda will be consid-ered one serving as people typically drink either size in one sitting.

Calories—larger type. This may be a design improvement, but that's about all. Remember, the quantity of calories is not as important as the *quality* of the calories, which you can only determine by reading the ingredients list.

Updated "Daily Values." The recommended daily values (DV) for sodium, dietary fiber, and vitamin D are changing slightly. According

to the FDA, they will be updated as follows, based on the latest scientific evidence:

Sodium: The general recommended daily limit for sodium will remain the same at 2,300 milligrams (which some experts believe is still too high), but it will extend to people older than age fifty and African Americans. Previously, these two demo-graphics were advised to limit their daily intake to 1,500 milligrams or less, which is now recommended only for those with hypertension or prehypertension. Note that the American Heart Association still advises all adults to keep sodium under 1,500 milli-grams a day.

Dietary fiber: This changes from a minimum of twenty-five grams to twenty-eight grams (which some experts believe is still low, but a definite improvement).

Vitamin D: The percent DV of vitamin D increases from 400 to 600 milligrams.

Nutrition Facts Panel Breakdown

Following are more specifics in each category to help you get the most information you can from the panel to make the healthiest food choices possible.

CALORIES

The number of calories alone doesn't give you enough information to make a smart decision about a food product. For example, Harvard researchers published a study in the *Journal of the American Medical Association* that found that eating a low glycemic diet, one that keeps blood sugar stable by avoiding sugar and simple carbohydrates (such as white bread or other refined foods), leads to a more ideal weight and better health compared to a low-fat or low-carb diet—even when the total calories were the same.

Other research, as mentioned elsewhere in this book, has shown that when calorie counts were equal, people who included nuts or fruit in their diets lost more weight.

These studies, and others like them, fiercely challenge the notion that "a calorie is a calorie."

For calories, the more important factor is their source. Low glycemic, whole food sources, such as vegetables, legumes, whole grains, nuts, and seeds, provide high-quality calories. Consumption of these foods is associated with a healthier weight, less inflammation, and less chronic disease.

Sugar-rich and refined foods (bread, pasta, pretzels, etc.) contain low-quality calories, and the consumption of such foods is associated with weight gain, inflammation, and more chronic disease.

Even if you were to eat the same number of calories of each, they'd affect your body in very different ways, and the outcome would be a body that looks and feels very different. *This is why the ingredients list is the most important part of a label.*

PERCENT DAILY VALUE (DV)

The percent DV indicates how much one serving of food contributes to the daily recommended intake of a nutrient. It is based on a 2,000-calorie diet for a healthy adult.

TOTAL FAT

Your body needs fat for a variety of reasons, so severely restricting it is unnecessary. And if weight loss is what you're after, restricting fat certainly isn't the best way to go. In the Harvard study published in the *Journal of the American Medical Association* mentioned previously, the low-fat diet was associated

with the least potential for weight loss as well as an unhealthy lipid pattern and increased insulin resistance. Meanwhile, a small human study published in the *International Journal of Obesity* found that when calories were equal, obese dieters who skimp on fat are more likely to develop gallstones than those who don't.

Don't fear fat! We need fat to absorb fat-soluble vitamins, keep our skin healthy, cushion our organs, regulate our body temperature, and provide energy. Fat is also necessary for the production of steroid hormones, including estrogen and testosterone, so restricting it may cause hormonal imbalances, particularly in women.

What's more, when fat is removed from a product that naturally contains it—such as dairy, for example—some sort of filler, typically sugar or salt, is added to make it palatable—and that's worse. Ditch the processed low-fat and no-fat products for good.

TRANS FATS

Trans fats are extremely harmful manmade fats used in packaged products to extend their shelf life. Although they've been in use since the 1950s, we now know they're inextricably linked with heart disease—the number one killer in America and globally. As of June 2015, the FDA has officially removed GRAS or "generally recognized as safe" status from trans fat and has given food manufacturers until June 2018 to eliminate it completely from their products. (Smaller food companies have until 2019 to comply.)

Until then, avoiding it is up to you. But this isn't as simple as reading the Nutrition Facts panel. Because of a labeling loophole, the front of a box and its Nutrition Facts panel are allowed to list a product as "0 grams trans fat"—when, in fact, one serving of the product can contain up to 0.5 grams of it. So, the only way to know if it's in your food is to read the ingredients list. If it contains any type of partially hydrogenated oil, the product contains trans fat—avoid it.

CHOLESTEROL

Cholesterol is found in animal-based products, such as meat and dairy, and is also made naturally in the body. For decades, we've been warned against eating foods high in cholesterol because they were thought to cause heart attacks, stroke, and other cardiovascular disease. The most recent research, though, shows us that cholesterol in food has little effect on cholesterol in the bloodstream (which is made by the body)—and that's the cholesterol that matters.

According to the scientific advisory panel for the 2015 iteration of the *Dietary Guidelines for Americans*, "Cholesterol is not a nutrient of concern for overconsumption." It turns out that sugar is more likely to cause heart attacks than eggs. A rigorous study published in *JAMA Internal Medicine* followed forty thousand people and found those who had the highest intake of sugar had a 400 percent increase in their risk of heart attack—even more evidence that the amount of sugar on the Nutrition Facts panel is the most crucial piece of information listed there.

SODIUM

Sodium, a mineral, is essential for keeping your heartbeat steady, conducting nerve impulses, and maintaining the proper balance of water and minerals, among other vital functions. However, most Americans get much more sodium than they need, which can cause high blood pressure and, in turn, increase the risk of heart attack, stroke, and kidney disease. The salt typically found in packaged foods is non-iodized refined salt, which is chemically cleaned, bleached, and devoid of minerals and is best limited or avoided.

Although U.S. federal guidelines suggest an upper limit of one teaspoon (6 g) per day, the American Heart Association recommends a maximum of two-thirds of a teaspoon (4 g) per day. The average American consumes at least one and a half teaspoons (9 g) per day, far more than our bodies need.

POTASSIUM

Potassium is an essential mineral, vital to the proper functioning of the cardiac, skeletal, and gastrointestinal systems. Because it's found in so many foods, most people get adequate amounts. However, if you consume too much sodium, it is possible to become potassium deficient because the more sodium you consume, the more potassium your body excretes.

TOTAL CARBOHYDRATES

This number refers to the combined amount of starch, sugar, and fiber in a product. Don't be scared of carbohydrates—your body needs them to function properly, and a low- or no-carb diet has been associated with increased cortisol levels, which can lead to insulin resistance and higher C-reactive protein levels, which may also increase risk of cardiovascular disease.

Not all carbs are created equal, though. For good health, avoid or eliminate refined carbs, including refined sugar and white flour. However, carbs from vegetables, fruit, grains, and legumes are good for you. Ideally, you want to consume carbs as close to their whole forms as possible because the more refined they are, the higher glycemic they are (yet another reason the Nutrition Facts panel alone is not enough). For example, brown rice (whole food form) is lower glycemic than brown rice flour (refined form), and steel cut oats (whole food form) are lower glycemic than instant oats (refined form).

DIETARY FIBER

Fiber is a complex carbohydrate that's an important part of the diet—yet most Americans consume far too little. Fiber is only found in plant-based foods and is often absent or minimal in packaged foods. It maintains bowel regularity and also decreases your risk for obesity, type 2 diabetes, high cholesterol, and colorectal cancer.

Your body can't digest fiber, so it doesn't provide energy or affect blood sugar levels. Basically, fiber acts like a broom, sweeping out your colon. Choose products that are naturally high in fiber to support digestion, keep you feeling satisfied longer, and help prevent disease.

SUGAR

Sugar is a simple carbohydrate that's digested quickly and used for energy. There are two sources of sugar: naturally occurring sugars (for example, in fruit or vegetables) and added refined sugar (often found in packaged and prepared foods). The current Nutrition Facts panel does not distinguish between the two, which is another reason to check the ingredients list first, as they both have different consequences for the body. In fact, your body doesn't need refined sugar at all. It offers no benefits (other than energy from calories) and only increases your risk for many types of disease and weight gain. But naturally occurring sugar, such as the sugar in fruit, is balanced with the fruit's beneficial fiber and nutrients, making naturally sweet foods a superior choice.

Interestingly, you'll notice there is not currently a percent DV for sugar on the panel. This is because, until recently, there was no federal guideline on sugar, as there are for other nutrients on the panel. And this has been convenient for manufacturers because just one serving of many products—including "healthy" foods, such as yogurt—would exceed the maximum recommended amount of twenty-five grams per day, a figure set by the American Heart Association.

Robert Lustig, M.D., a pediatric endocrinologist at the University of California, who cites its inextricable link to our nation's rise in obesity and many types of disease, goes so far as to say we shouldn't be consuming refined sugar at all.

The updated Nutrition Facts panel will feature a percent DV for sugar: However, at fifty grams of sugar a day for someone consuming a two-thousand-calorie diet, it's double what the American Heart Association recommends as an absolute maximum. For optimum health, aim for fewer than twenty-five grams of added sugar a day—or, for the new percent DV on the new labels, up to 50 percent DV daily.

PROTEIN

Protein is a necessary nutrient, but in addition to the amount, look for the source, which you'll find in the ingredients list. In packaged products, such as snacks or meal bars, look for plant-based sources, such as nuts, seeds, peas, or grains. They're a superior choice to animal-based sources, such as whey, dairy, or meat, which are typically less health supportive, more calorie dense, and not organic. (For the full scoop on why choosing organic animal products is crucial, see chapters 8 and 11.) The one exception to this rule is soy protein. Processed soy, often seen in the ingredients list as soy protein isolate, is controversial and best avoided. See chapter 6 for more details.

VITAMINS & MINERALS

Vitamins and minerals are a critical part of our diets; they're necessary for normal body function and good health. Most Nutrition Facts panels only show four nutrients: vitamin A, vitamin C, calcium, and iron as well as their recommended percent DVs. The new panel will replace vitamins A and C with vitamin D and potassium.

In truth, our bodies need at least thirteen necessary vitamins, sixteen minerals, and hundreds—if not thousands—of antioxidants and phytochemicals. All these vitamins and minerals are available to us through food—but not just any food. They're mainly found in whole foods. (Note there are limited food sources of vitamin D. Our bodies create vitamin D when exposed to the sun.)

While some processed foods do contain vitamins, they're often fortified, which means the natural vitamins and minerals were stripped out initially (for example, in white bread or cereal) and synthetic vitamins were then added (which you'll see in the ingredients list). Synthetic vitamins are inferior to naturally occurring ones, and, in fact, some can be toxic when consumed in large amounts, such as vitamins A and E. The best sources of vitamins, minerals, antioxidants, and phytochemicals are the fresh, unprocessed foods that don't come with a Nutrition Facts panel.

Final Thoughts on the Nutrition Facts Panel

In light of the preceding inadequacies, the Nutrition Facts panel gives an incomplete picture of the healthiness of a food. Currently, the amount of sugar per serving is the line item with which you should be most concerned. While the new 2018 label is an improvement, the source of the calories—that is, the ingredients—will always be the best indicator of a product's health value. Always read the ingredients list first!

Ingredients List

If you feel like you need a degree in food science to figure out what's in your favorite packaged food, you're not alone. Part of the reason people glaze over the ingredients list stems from the fact they can't understand it.

There are increasing numbers of ingredients synthesized in laboratories, and while they may have desirable effects for food manufacturers (such as more attractive colors or flavors, extended shelf life, or increased profits), many have not-so-desirable effects on our health.

So when determining the health value of any packaged food, look first to the ingredients list. The rest of this chapter explains why you should avoid certain ingredients or types of foods. The following chapters then provide concrete guidelines for reading the ingredients list and choosing the healthiest versions of just about any type of packaged food.

Twelve Controversial Ingredients to Avoid

WARNING! This section is downright scary (at least to me). Though I've managed to almost completely avoid these controversial ingredients over the past eight years, my belly was a controversial-ingredient garbage dump for the previous two decades. I ate every single one of them—and frequently, which is probably why I ended up fat, sick, and lethargic by the age of eighteen. The good news, though, is that I didn't die. I'm still here—and I'm doing great now.

So, if you realize some of your favorite foods contain the scary little buggers on this list, don't freak out. Just go through your cabinets and throw out the foods that contain them. Replace them with healthier swaps, as outlined in the coming chapters. And move on.

Vow not to buy food that will harm your health from this point forward. Now you know; before, you didn't. No use crying over spilled almond milk.

Plus, these twelve controversial ingredients are so commonly used in packaged foods that it would almost be *more* strange if you *weren't* currently consuming any. And you don't need to memorize them—all but two fall into the "ingredients you would not stock in your own kitchen" category—which, as you'll learn in the next chapter, should be avoided anyway.

Fasten your seat belt. Here's the scary truth about what you've been eating.

ASPARTAME & ARTIFICIAL SWEETENERS

Artificial sweeteners make foods sweet without the calories of sugar, making them a popular choice for any sort of "diet" food. But, they come at a cost, and I bet you'd rather take regular sugar—calories and all—once you see the price tag.

In a 1996 *60 Minutes* episode, correspondent Mike Wallace stated that aspartame's approval in 1981 was "the most contested in FDA history." At the time, independent studies found that it caused brain cancer in lab animals, and the studies submitted for FDA approval by G.D. Searle, the manufacturer of aspartame, were flawed. Former Senator Howard Metzenbaum is quoted in the interview as saying: "According to the FDA themselves, Searle, when making their presentation to the FDA, had willfully misrepresented the facts, and withheld some of the facts they knew would possibly jeopardize the approval."

Consumers have reported dozens of adverse reactions to aspartame—from headaches to memory loss to seizures. Aspartame is believed to cause oxidative stress and neurodegeneration (destruction of brain cells).

Artificial sweeteners can also disrupt blood sugar and increase hunger. (The paradox of diet food is that the more you eat of it, the more weight you typically gain.)

It is most commonly found in diet foods, diet drinks, sugar-free desserts, candy, and various confections.

ARTIFICIAL COLORS

Other names: FD&C Blue No. 1, FD&C Blue No. 2, FD&C Green No. 3, FD&C Red No. 40, FD&C Red No. 3, FD&C Yellow No. 5, FD&C Yellow No. 6

Artificial colors look pretty and that is, indeed, their sole purpose—to make food more visually appealing. Back in the old days, we used fruit and vegetable juices or spices to color food, but these artificial colors come from petroleum. The FDA maintains they're safe: However, a growing body of evidence has linked them to behavioral problems in children. The Center for Science in the Public Interest has petitioned the FDA to ban artificial food dyes because of this.

After a 2007 British study showed that artificial colors increased hyperactivity in children, products sold in Britain that contain any one of the six food dyes studied must bear the statement, "may have an adverse effect on activity and attention in children." These include Yellow 5, Yellow 6, Red 3, and Red 40 and two dyes not used in the United States. Though the dyes were not outlawed, many manufacturers voluntarily switched to more natural dyes to avoid putting that statement on their packages.

Beyond behavioral problems, some of the dyes are known or suspected carcinogens. For example, Red 3 was recognized by the FDA as a thyroid carcinogen in animals and is banned in cosmetics and externally applied drugs, but is still allowed in food and internal drugs. Red 40, the most widely used dye, may accelerate the appearance of immune system tumors in mice. Based on this limited, yet growing, body of research, you may want to think twice about feeding your kids (or yourself) artificial food dyes.

These dyes are most commonly found in baked goods, candy, cereal, chips, snack foods, sports drinks, yogurts, and anything brightly or darkly colored, including the brown crust on some white bread or the brown "chocolate-like" substance that covers candy bars.

ARTIFICIAL FLAVORS

With all the delicious varieties of natural foods, it's mind-boggling that we humans created artificial flavors in the first place. Humans are hardwired to like certain flavors, such as the sweetness of fruit or the saltiness of celery, and to reject others—anything that tastes too bitter, which could signal poison.

Because packaged food is so heavily processed and refined, if it weren't for salt, sugar, fat, or flavoring agents, they wouldn't have much taste at all. Plus, added flavoring agents make products taste fresh—even though they're months old. But artificial flavors aren't just used to make food palatable: They're sometimes used to make it addictive, too. In a 2011 *60 Minutes* interview, correspondent Morley Safer interviewed two food scientists from Givaudan, the dominant player in flavor and fragrance creation for food companies. The scientists described how they make fruit flavors—such as the ones in breakfast cereals and snack foods—that yield a burst of flavor at first, but don't linger for long. Why? Because "you're not going to eat more if it lingers," both scientists said. Safer follows up with a clarification: "But that suggests something else . . . which is addiction." "Exactly,"

one of the food scientists replies. "That's a good word."

The term "artificial flavors" can be used for hundreds of different synthetic chemicals, many of which are derived from petroleum. They're often used in inferior junk food, as they offer no nutritive value—just flavor, at a lower cost than real, natural ingredients. Because you have no idea which artificial flavors you're getting, this can be a concern for people who have uncommon food allergies or are on a restricted diet. They've been linked to allergic reactions, dermatitis, eczema, hyperactivity, and asthma.

Artificial flavors are most commonly found in beverages, candy, cereals, mac and cheese, snack foods, and yogurts.

BROMINATED VEGETABLE OIL (BVO)

Brominated vegetable oil doesn't sound too bad; after all, it has the word "vegetable" in it. But it's not nearly as innocuous as it seems. This additive, which is used to keep flavor oils in suspension throughout a liquid, is banned in more than 100 countries (not including the United States) because it's linked to thyroid issues, autoimmune issues, reproductive interference, and birth defects. After intense consumer petitioning in 2014, both Coca-Cola and PepsiCo vowed to remove BVO from their U.S. products, and while they've removed it from some products—such as Gatorade and Powerade—it remains in others. And neither company has provided a timeline for full removal of BVO from all their products.

BVO is most commonly found in soft drinks and sports drinks.

BUTYLATED HYDROXYANISOLE (BHA) & BUTYLATED HYDROXYTOLUENE (BHT)

BHA and BHT are preservatives that prevent oils and animal fat from going rancid. At a minimum, they have been linked to a weakened immune system, but, at worst, they've been linked to disrupting the nervous system, the endocrine system, and behavior. Plus, they're suspected carcinogens that may lower sperm and egg production.

Although both are designated as GRAS, the National Toxicology Program classifies BHA as "reasonably anticipated to be a human carcinogen." BHA is also listed as a known carcinogen under California's Proposition 65, a list that contains a wide range of naturally occurring and synthetic chemicals known to cause cancer or birth defects or other reproductive harm.

BHA and BHT are most commonly found in beer, butter, cake, chips, cookies, gum, meat, microwaveable dinners, sausage, and vegetable oil.

MONOSODIUM GLUTAMATE (MSG)

Other names: torula yeast, yeast extract, autolyzed yeast extract, malted barley, textured whey protein, hydrolyzed vegetable protein

Food manufacturers love MSG. It may trick your body into wanting to eat more, which almost guarantees you'll keep going back to buy more.

A study published in the *American Journal of Clinical Nutrition*, which followed more than ten thousand adults for an average of five and a half years, found that people who eat more MSG are more likely to be overweight or obese. Participants who ate the most MSG were 30 percent more likely to become overweight by the end of the study.

The link between MSG and weight gain isn't entirely clear. Some experts speculate that because the food tastes good, people want more of it. Others, such as the authors of this study, think it may have something to do with the hormone leptin, which regulates appetite and metabolism. They found that MSG may cause leptin resistance, which may explain why people who ate more MSG gained more weight, regardless of how many calories they consumed.

Aside from weight gain, MSG has been linked to headaches, itchy skin, dizziness, sweating, numbness, tingling or burning sensations, flushing, heart palpitations, nausea, chest pain, and weakness.

MSG is most commonly found in canned vegetables, frozen entrées, fast foods, and snack foods including chips and meal bars.

NATURAL FLAVORS

If you're like me, when you hear the world "natural," you immediately conjure up images of rolling fields, vibrant flowers, and a bubbling brook. But add the word "flavors" to it and all of a sudden, I'm thinking beaver butt. Natural flavors do, at least, come from a real plant or animal source instead of a lab. But, remember, a gland in a beaver's anus counts as "natural," too. And no, I'm not kidding. For instance, that's where the natural flavor castoreum comes from, which is used as a substitute for vanilla flavor. Although synthetic vanillin, which mostly comes from petrochemicals, is much more widely used (about 300 pounds, or 136 kg, of castoreum are consumed annually, in comparison with more than 2.6 million pounds, or 1.2 million kg, of synthetic vanillin), this example demonstrates that you don't really know what you're getting when a company uses a vague umbrella term such as this one.

"Natural flavors" could mean one flavor or a combination of hundreds of different things—some of which you'd probably rather not eat, such as the aforementioned animal secretion as well as BHA or propylene glycol, the main ingredient in antifreeze. And because the term sounds so innocent, it's also a good place to sneak in chemicals that can manipulate the appetite.

Natural flavors are most commonly found in cereals, meal bars, orange juice, snack foods, and yogurt.

NITRATE & NITRITE

These two common preservatives are added to deli meat to allow it to retain its color and flavor and to keep it from being spoiled by bacterial growth. The World Health Organization has declared them to be probable human carcinogens. One study, published in the *Journal of the National Cancer Institute*, followed more than 190,000 people, ages forty-five to seventy-five, for seven years, and found that the people who consumed the most processed meat had a 67 percent higher risk of pancreatic cancer than those who ate the least amount.

These two common preservatives are most commonly found in cured meats such as bacon, salami, ham, sausage, hot dogs, bologna, pepperoni, and other deli meats.

PARTIALLY HYDROGENATED OILS/TRANS FAT

Other names: Trans fat, partially hydrogenated vegetable oil, partially hydrogenated soybean oil, partially hydrogenated cottonseed oil, etc.

First introduced to the American food supply as shortening in 1911, the effects of trans fat started coming into question as early as 1956, right before the FDA automatically grandfathered it in as an ingredient generally recognized as safe (GRAS) for the food supply. Research criticizing trans fats picked up in the 1990s, with multiple studies linking it to cardiovascular disease. By 2009, cardiac disease researcher Fred Kummerow, Ph.D., got tired of waiting for the FDA to do its job, so he petitioned the FDA to ban trans fat based on the uncontested evidence of its harmful health effects. Six months later, he filed a lawsuit against the FDA after it failed to respond within a reasonable period of time. That woke up the FDA—but it continued to plod on at a glacial pace. Meanwhile, the Centers for Disease Control and Prevention published a report in 2012 that estimated that up to twenty thousand heart attacks and seven thousand cardiac deaths each year are caused by consumption of trans fat.

In November 2013, the FDA finally issued a statement that there was enough evidence to suggest that no amount of trans fat is safe for human consumption. In June 2015, nearly two years after questioning its GRAS status, the FDA finalized its decision and has given food manufacturers three years to remove trans fats from their products.

So, by June 2018, nine years after the initial lawsuit was filed, trans fat will no longer be permitted for use in food products. But you do have to look out for it until then, and—even more maddeningly—it's often hidden. Thanks to a labeling loophole, a package can say it contains no trans fat—when, in fact, one serving can contain up to 0.5 grams of the stuff. (And we all know plenty of packages that appear to be one individual serving often actually contain two or three servings, according to the nutrition panel.) The only surefire way to avoid it is to read the ingredients list and avoid anything with partially hydrogenated oil.

Trans fat is most commonly found in snack foods, microwave popcorn, crackers, croissants, and any baked products in a package.

POTASSIUM BROMATE

The recipe for bread is wheat, water, and yeast. It's pretty hard to mess that up. But leave it to food manufacturers to get crafty in the kitchen (read: lab) and add some modern chemicals to speed up production and lower costs (for them, anyway). Potassium bromate is a chemical used to strengthen bread and cracker dough and help it rise during baking. Unfortunately for the consumer, this chemical has been linked to a variety of concerns, including an increased toxin load for your kidneys, DNA damage, and even cancer.

If you get your bread and baked goods from a real bakery, you shouldn't have to worry about it. But be on the lookout for this on any packaged baked products.

This chemical is most commonly found in baked goods, particularly bread, crackers, and chips.

PROPYL PARABEN

If you're familiar with the word "paraben," it's probably from shopping the (natural) beauty aisle, where you'll see lotions, shampoos, and toothpaste proudly sporting the label, "paraben free." But this chemical hasn't been banished completely: It not only remains in thousands of beauty products, but also in food.

Propyl paraben is used as a preservative in tortillas and other baked goods. And available data suggest that parabens act as estrogenic endocrine disruptors, which means they can wreak havoc on your hormones. Animal studies have linked them to decreased testosterone levels in males; test tube studies have linked them to the proliferation of human breast cancer cells; and human studies have linked them to fertility issues in women. Clearly, this is an ingredient you can do without, and it's easy to avoid—as long as you read the ingredients list. (While you're at it, it's probably a good idea to avoid it in your cosmetics and natural care products, too!)

Propyl paraben is most commonly found in baked goods, beverages, dairy products, muffins, and tortillas.

REFINED SUGAR

Other names: raw sugar, white sugar, table sugar, brown sugar, evaporated cane juice, cane sugar, corn syrup, high fructose corn syrup, fruit juice concentrate, maltose, dextrose, sucrose

You may wonder how little ol' table sugar made its way onto this big, bad list. Surprisingly, it's perhaps the most consumed—and controversial—of them all.

Sugar is everywhere, even in surprising places like tomato sauce, savory salad dressing, and bread. Manufacturers love adding it to everything because it lights up pleasure sensors in the brain, making us desire, and even crave, their products. And, of course, it's cheap. Its usage is much more widespread than any of the other chemicals on this list.

There are many problems with sugar. To start, sugar promotes weight gain. With the way our bodies metabolize it, it gets stored as fat quite readily. So it's no surprise it's considered one of the main culprits behind our obesity epidemic.

One of the risks of obesity is diabetes, and for a long time, it was thought that sugar only contributed indirectly to diabetes risk (because it promotes weight gain and obesity). However, a large epidemiological study that assessed 175 populations across the world during the past decade found that increased sugar in a population's food supply was linked to higher diabetes rates, independent of obesity rates. This doesn't prove sugar causes diabetes, but more sugar was correlated with more diabetes, and diabetes rates dropped when sugar availability dropped. This does suggest that sugar calories affect the liver and pancreas in ways other calories do not.

Also, sugar increases blood pressure and cholesterol levels, which may lead to more

Why Are These Controversial Ingredients Allowed in Our Food Supply Anyway?

You're probably wondering how it's even possible that ingredients such as these, either known or suspected to cause bodily harm, are allowed in the food supply in the first place.

The U.S. governmental agency that oversees the food supply—the Food and Drug Administration (FDA)—is technically supposed to act like border control, either rejecting or allowing ingredients into the food supply. Since 1958, the FDA has kept a list of ingredients allowed to be used in food products, called the "generally recognized as safe" (GRAS) list.

Any ingredients in use prior to 1958 were automatically added to the list based on "experience of their common use in food." Essentially, if an ingredient had been used in food until that point without major concern, it was assumed to be safe and was grandfathered in without any scientific testing. As hindsight shows us, dozens of these additives turned out to be dangerous or downright deadly. In 1970, after the artificial sweetener cyclamate was found to cause liver tumors in rats and its GRAS status was revoked, the public started to question all the new-fangled ingredients showing up in packaged foods. So President Richard Nixon ordered the FDA to reevaluate the GRAS list using scientific standards. By 1982, a scientific committee had evaluated four hundred substances: thirty were recommended for removal, and five were flagged for raised safety concerns. Despite this, the FDA reaffirmed the GRAS status of seventeen of these ingredients and never did anything with the others.

Any ingredients introduced after 1958 were supposed to be subject to scientific scrutiny before being allowed on the market. Here's how that worked: Between 1958 and 1997, the manufacturer of an ingredient would hire a panel of expert scientists to undertake research on the safety of its product and then petition the FDA on its behalf. The FDA would review the scientific information provided by the company and either affirm it as GRAS or ask for more research. This wasn't ideal, as a company that funded scientific research for its own product could pose a conflict of interest, but the situation got even worse.

In 1997, the FDA proposed that manufacturers and trade groups determine whether their ingredients would qualify as GRAS. The FDA didn't wait for its proposal to become a rule. It adopted it, and this procedure is still in effect today, essentially letting the food industry police itself. If the manufacturer so chooses, it can have the FDA review and affirm its self-determined GRAS status.

Between 2004 and 2010, only fourteen food additive petitions were sent to the FDA. During that same period, 222 ingredients received GRAS status by self-determination. In essence, the FDA has outsourced its main function to the food industry, which now polices and regulates itself. With its history of lax standards and current lack of personnel and funding, it's not surprising that potentially dangerous chemicals end up on our grocery store shelves.

There is hope, though. You can easily avoid these ingredients simply by getting into the habit of reading ingredients lists. Anytime you pick up a box, flip it over—period.

And, if what you just learned makes your blood boil, don't stay silent. Consider supporting one of these four groups working to fix the broken U.S. food system: the Center for Science in the Public Interest; Consumers Union; the Environmental Working Group; and Natural Resources Defense Council.

serious heart health issues, such as heart disease, the number one cause of death globally. It promotes inflammation in the body, which can lead to other more serious health conditions, and has also been found to impair cognitive function, including learning ability and memory.

Okay, I know I've just crushed your guilty pleasure. But wait—there's hope. You can still eat sweet things. (Yes, even the occasional cookie or cake!) It just pays to be smart about it. Ideally, you should choose items made with more gentle natural sweeteners, as outlined in chapter 13. I promise they taste just as good, if not better, than refined sugar.

Refined sugar is most commonly found in your pantry as well as almost anything and everything in a package, including sweets, crackers, cereal, desserts, salad dressings, tomato sauce, bread, and more.

Genetically Modified Foods (GMO)

Of all the controversial food ingredients, none stirs up quite such a heated debate as GMOs. While any organism—including plants, viruses, animals, and bacteria—could be GMO, the ones that make it into our food supply have caused the biggest uproar.

At its simplest, a GMO food crop has had its genetic material artificially manipulated to give it a specific trait or to cause it to grow in a more desirable way that does not occur in nature.

FDA approval for GMOs is based on scientific research provided by the very biotech companies that created them—without any third-party testing. Apparently, this research was enough to convince the FDA that GMOs are not substantially different or unique compared to conventional crops. However, those same biotech companies also went to the United States Patent and Trademark Office and were able to score patents on these very same crops based on the assertion they're substantially different and unique compared to conventional crops. Go figure.

WHY DO GMOS EXIST?

GMOs were introduced into the American food supply in 1998 under the impression they'd achieve two things: increase crop yields to increase farmers' efficiency and profitability and decrease pesticide use by creating crops that contain "intrinsic pesticides."

GMOs are also sometimes used to create more nutrient-dense foods—although malnutrition isn't as great a concern in America as it is in other countries, so it can be assumed that the preceding two reasons were the driving forces behind our adoption of GMOs.

ARE GMOS SAFE?

According to the companies that created them, such as Monsanto and DuPont, yes, GMOs are safe. However, there have been no independent, large, long-term, human studies that confirm the safety of human consumption of GMOs. There are a number of small, independent, human and animal studies, though, that do raise concerns over the health risks associated with GMO consumption, including adverse effects on the liver, pancreas, kidneys, blood, and reproductive organs. Large, long-term studies are expensive, and no one has coughed up the funds to pay for them—but that doesn't mean the risks aren't there.

At the bare minimum, even if GMO crops themselves don't harm health, glyphosate—the herbicide they're treated with—probably does. The World Health Organization recently classified glyphosate as a probable human carcinogen. It's also connected to gastrointestinal issues, nutritional deficiencies, autism, Alzheimer's, and cardiovascular disease.

Regardless of health concerns—and most perplexingly—federal reports indicate that during the past fifteen years of use, GMOs have not lived up to the purported goals for which they were created. In 2014, the U.S. Department of Agriculture's Economic Research Service published a report based on the results of GMO seed use from 1998 to 2013 that stated: "Over the first fifteen years of commercial use, genetically engineered seeds have not been shown to definitively increase yield potentials . . . in fact, the yields of herbicide-tolerant or insect-resistant seeds may be occasionally lower than yields of conventional varieties."

As far as chemical spraying goes, according to an independent study published in 2012 in the journal *Environmental Sciences Europe*, "Herbicide-resistant crop technology has led to a 239 million kilogram (527 million pounds) increase in herbicide use in the United States between 1996 and 2011, while insect-resistant crops have reduced insecticide applications by fifty-six million kilograms (123 million pounds). Overall, pesticide use increased by an estimated 183 million kilograms (403 million pounds), or about 7 percent."

ARE GMOs LABELED?

GMOs are not labeled in the United States, thanks in no small part to the powerful biotech lobby, which has helped thwart any regulation that would require it. Most people aren't even aware they're eating them. In more than sixty countries, though, including all of Europe, Australia, and Japan, there are significant restrictions—or outright bans—on the production and sale of GMOs. At the minimum, manufacturers must label foods that contain GMOs clearly so consumers can decide whether to consume them.

So, how can we avoid GMOs? Currently, the most common GMO foods available in the United States are the following:

- Alfalfa
- Canola
- Corn
- Papaya
- Soy
- Sugar beets
- Zucchini and yellow summer squash

You can safely assume any of these foods in their conventional forms are GMO, as GMO crops comprise between 88 and 95 percent of U.S. crops. Plus, in February 2015, the FDA approved GMO apples (Arctic apples) and GMO potatoes (Innate) that resist bruising and don't brown when cut. This means they'll probably make it to a grocery store near you in the coming years.

Don't forget that these crops are often used in packaged foods as well. According to the Grocery Manufacturers Association, as much as 80 percent of packaged foods contain GMO ingredients, such as beet sugar or derivatives of corn, soy, or canola. Following is a table that lists all their derivatives, which will give you an idea of how pervasive these GMO ingredients are.

To avoid GMOs, look for the USDA Organic or Non-GMO Project Verified seal on foods or packaged products that contain the common GMO ingredients.

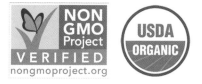

Also, keep in mind that you can be exposed to GMOs through meat because livestock on conventional meat farms are often fed GMO alfalfa and corn. Organic livestock are not fed GMOs, however.

Canned Foods

Canned foods make our lives infinitely easier, but they may not always be the best choice. Most metal food cans contain a chemical called bisphenol A, more commonly known as BPA. It's an endocrine disruptor and can be particularly harmful to babies in the womb or in early life. Chronic exposure to BPA has been associated with serious health problems, including heart disease and cancer.

According to a study published in *Hypertension*, a journal of the American Heart Association, even a single exposure, such as one glass of soy milk from a BPA-lined container, has a direct and immediate effect on cardiovascular health: It raises blood pressure in just a few hours. Although an isolated episode of elevated blood pressure isn't much cause for alarm, if you're constantly consuming foods contaminated with BPA, you may be at a higher risk for hypertension.

The FDA banned the use of BPA in baby bottles, sippy cups, and infant formulas, but it remains in many metal food cans. Based on the associated ill effects of BPA and on consumer concern, some manufacturers voluntarily started using BPA-free cans. However, the most recent research shows that the most common alternatives, BPC and BPS, are just as toxic—or even more toxic—than BPA.

So, the wisest choice may be to skip canned goods altogether. Instead, choose glass packages, frozen packages, fresh foods, or dry goods.

🅖 **Money-Saving Tip**

Skip canned beans and cook your own for a healthier, truly BPA-free, and less expensive alternative. Though the beans have to soak at least overnight before cooking (see page 134), your time in the kitchen is minimal. The simplest way is to invest in a pressure cooker (usually around $100), which will cook your presoaked beans in a matter of minutes instead of hours. Freshly cooked beans are not only more nutritious, they're more delicious as well! Plus, beans freeze well and thaw quickly, so don't be afraid to make a big batch.

Hidden GMO Sources in Packaged Foods

Unless organic or Non-GMO verified, the following ingredients may be GMO:

Aspartame	Glutamic acid	Mono and diglycerides
Baking powder	Glycerides	Monosodium glutamate (MSG)
Canola oil (rapeseed oil)	Glycine	Shoyu
Caramel color	Hemicellulose	Sorbitol
Cellulose	High fructose corn syrup (HFCS)	Soy flour
Citric acid	Hydrogenated starch	Soy isolates
Cobalamin (vitamin B_{12})	Hydrolyzed vegetable protein	Soy lecithin
Condensed milk	Inverse syrup	Soy milk
Confectioners' sugar	Invert sugar	Soy oil
Corn flour	Lactic acid	Soy protein
Corn masa	Lecithin	Soy protein isolate
Corn meal	Leucine	Soy sauce
Corn oil	Lysine	Starch
Corn sugar	Maltitol	Stearic acid
Corn syrup	Malt	Sugar (unless specified as cane sugar)
Cornstarch	Malt syrup	Tamari
Cottonseed oil	Malt extract	Tempeh
Dextrin	Oleic acid	Teriyaki marinades
Glycerin	Phenylalanine	Textured vegetable protein
Glycerol	Phytic acid	Threonine
Dextrose	Protein isolate	Tocopherols (vitamin E)
Diacetyl	Maltodextrin	Tofu
Diglyceride	Maltose	Trehalose
Erythritol	Mannitol	Triglyceride
Food starch	Methylcellulose	Vegetable fat
Fructose (any form)	Milk powder	Vegetable oil
Glucose	Modified food starch	Whey
Glutamate	Modified starch	Xanthan gum

CHAPTER 13

PANTRY STAPLES

Navigating the packaged food aisles can be tricky. The following pages are here to help. This chapter shows you how to choose the healthiest versions of a wide variety of pantry staples—and how to ditch the food imposters. (If you've read Chapters 4 through 11, these recommendations will make sense. If you have questions, return to the relevant chapter for more information.)

These general guidelines will empower you to make the best decisions when it comes to packaged foods. If you're interested in specific brand recommendations, head to mariamarlowe.com/real-food-guide.

To get started, here are the top five tips for selecting the healthiest packaged foods:

1. **Avoid any ingredients you wouldn't stock in your own kitchen.** This is usually the unpronounceable stuff, but also includes things such as "high fructose corn syrup" or "natural flavors."

2. **Avoid anything that lists sugar as the first or second ingredient.** Ingredients are listed by weight from highest to lowest, so if sugar is the first ingredient in a product, it contains more sugar than anything else. Sugar is linked with myriad health problems (see chapter 13); it's best to avoid it.

3. **Avoid anything with partially hydrogenated oils.** This is an indication of the presence of trans fat, a substance conclusively linked to heart attacks and cardiac deaths, even in small amounts.

4. **Avoid anything with inferior, inflammatory, or GMO oils.** These include soybean oil, corn oil, vegetable oil, palm oil, and rice bran oil. (To learn more about the best and worst oils see pages 224 to 231.)

5. **Avoid GMO ingredients.** Avoid foods that contain conventional corn, soy, canola, or any of their derivatives. Though tip number one on this list should cover most of them, see the full list of derivatives on page 212.

Specific Selection Guidelines by Food Type

Consider the following as you stock your pantry with healthy staples.

BROTH

Look for products that only contain water, vegetables or organic meats, and spices.

Watch out for sneaky ingredients such as sugar, carrageenan, and other additives, even in "healthy"-sounding brands.

Grains Classified

Watch out for Grains with Gluten	Look for Naturally Gluten-Free Grains
Barley	Amaranth
Bulgur	Buckwheat
Durum	Millet
Farro	Oats
Kamut	Quinoa
Pumpernickel	Rice
Rye	Sorghum
Semolina	Teff
Spelt	
Triticale	
Wheat	

BREAD

Look for gluten-free, sourdough, or sprouted breads that are either freshly baked or frozen. When you buy bread from a bakery, it goes stale the next day. When you buy bread from the grocery store, it can stay "fresh" for weeks or even months—thanks to preservatives, some of which are linked to health concerns. Instead look for baked goods without preservatives at the grocery store. These are typically found in the refrigerator or freezer section. Or buy your bread from a real bakery.

Watch out for baked goods with ingredients you wouldn't stock in your own kitchen, such as potassium bromate, azodicarbonamide, partially hydrogenated oil, monoglycerides and diglycerides, and butylated hydroxyanisole (BHA).

Gluten Intolerance

Humans have been eating bread for centuries. So why, all of a sudden, can't some people tolerate the gluten in it? Bread making dates back as far as the ancient Egyptians, who were the first to discover that adding yeast to grains made them rise. This technique was used for thousands of years. But this wasn't just any bread. It was sourdough—a type of bread made by a long dough-fermentation process using naturally occurring lactobacilli and yeast. Bread making changed only about 150 years ago, when commercial yeast was introduced. Now, bread can be made in three hours, instead of days or even weeks.

One theory explaining the increase in gluten intolerance claims it has nothing to do with the wheat, but everything to do with the process by which it's made. By eliminating the long fermentation process, we're skipping a key step that neutralizes the phytic acid naturally found in gluten and grains. When the phytic acid is left intact—as in modern breads—digestive troubles and allergic reactions may ensue. Though a little phytic acid may not be problematic, most Americans eat too much of it: a bagel for breakfast, a sandwich for lunch, and rolls at dinner, not to mention pretzels and crackers as snacks. Try switching to sourdough or sprouted breads and see whether you feel less bloated and heavy.

TORTILLAS

Look for those made with simple ingredients, such as brown rice, organic sprouted corn, or coconut flours: Find them in the refrigerator or freezer section because healthier tortillas don't contain preservatives.

Watch out for tortillas with ingredients such as potassium bromate, azodicarbonamide, partially hydrogenated oil, monoglycerides, diglycerides, and butylated hydroxyanisole (BHA).

⊚ Myth Alert!

Myth: Whole-wheat, whole-grain, or multi-grain bread is automatically healthy.

Fact: These types of breads may sound healthy, but, typically, they're not. The gluten in whole-wheat products can be inflammatory and cause digestive upset. Plus, most of these breads are loaded with preservatives, additives, and even white flour! Next time you're at the store, check your favorite bread's ingredients list. You may be surprised at what you find—artificial colors, multiple sweeteners, and chemical additives. What's more, most people are shocked to learn that a slice of whole-wheat toast will often raise your blood sugar more than a can of soda or a candy bar.

BAKING, COOKIE, PANCAKE & PIZZA MIXES

Look for a high-quality recipe you can make yourself to control the amount and types of sweeteners and other ingredients. Ideally, find a recipe that uses gluten-free flour or simply substitute it according to gluten-free flour package directions. In a pinch, look for gluten-free baking mixes with no added sugar (or minimal amounts).

Watch out for baking mixes that list sugar as the first or second ingredient or ones made with gluten-containing flour, such as wheat.

CEREAL & GRANOLA

Look for hot whole-grain cereals, such as oatmeal, quinoa, or buckwheat, as most cereal is pure sugar, wheat, and corn—the perfect trifecta for weight gain and poor health. For cold cereal and granola, look for sprouted gluten-free grains or Paleo-style cereals or granolas, which are made from nuts and seeds instead of grains.

Watch out for cereals with sugar as one of the top two ingredients, artificial colors, corn syrup, and added vitamins. Also, avoid instant or flavored oatmeal, which is less nutritious, higher glycemic, and often has added sugar.

CONDIMENTS

Look for ingredients that you would stock in your own kitchen.

Watch out for products with added sugar or too much sodium. More on specific condiments follows.

Horseradish

Horseradish contains more medicinally active compounds than most other spices. It can clear congestion and mucous, reduce inflammation, stimulate the immune system, and fight bacteria and viruses. Horseradish root is part of the cruciferous vegetable family, making it a source of glucosinolates, compounds being studied for their anticancer properties.

You may have had horseradish before. It's colored green with spinach and spirulina to make the wasabi paste served with sushi. It also turns ketchup into cocktail sauce. On its own, it's great with fish, eggs, baked beans, or in other homemade sauces. Horseradish is available in the refrigerated section. Look for a brand with minimal ingredients: horseradish, vinegar, and salt. Use the back of a fork to squeeze out as much vinegar as you can before adding it to food: That way, you get the full horseradish flavor.

❶ Expert Tip

Top your morning oats or buckwheat with cinnamon, fresh fruit, and nuts or seeds to make an ultra-filling, satisfying power breakfast that'll keep hunger at bay for hours.

Jam

Choose the brands lowest in sugar per serving and, ideally, choose organic as jam is typically made from fruit that's been heavily sprayed with pesticides. It's also easy to make your own.

Ketchup

Because ketchup is a tomato product, always choose organic to limit pesticide exposure and read the ingredients list to make sure that little to no sugar has been added.

Mayonnaise

Mayonnaise is an emulsion of oil, egg yolks, and vinegar. If you're going to eat it, choose an organic brand made with a high-quality oil, such as olive oil.

There are at least a few plant-based mayos on the market, and though they may taste like the real thing, they tend to be made from low-quality ingredients, such as canola oil and modified food starch, so they're best avoided or eaten in limited quantities.

Mustard

Mustard comes from the crucifer family, so it's no surprise it contains cancer-fighting compounds. It also contains anti-inflammatory omega-3 fats and may protect against certain types of cancer, including colon cancer.

There are three types of mustard. Yellow, found in American-style mustard, is the least pungent, which indicates it packs the smallest health punch, compared with the others. Brown mustard is slightly more pungent and can be found in spicy, brown, Dijon, and whole-grain mustards. Black is the most pungent and, therefore, the most potent. It can be found in whole-grain mustards.

Choose mustards with minimal to no added sugar and for the most health benefits, select whole-grain mustards.

Pickles

Naturally fermented pickles contain beneficial probiotics that promote a healthy digestive tract. Some commercial varieties are no longer traditionally fermented and use vinegar instead of salt: You won't get the same health benefits from these. Avoid any pickles with vinegar in the ingredients list and choose varieties with salt and and/or spices only. And don't think you have to stick only to pickled cucumbers! Any pickled vegetable will work, such as beets or carrots. For the freshest pickles, choose those in the refrigerator section.

Sauerkraut & Kimchi

Sauerkraut is pickled or fermented cabbage. When made traditionally, it contains those beneficial probiotics that aid a healthy digestive tract. Kimchi is the spicy Korean version of pickled vegetables. Both are great additions to your diet, supporting digestive health.

Salad Dressings

Skip bottled salad dressings: They're often loaded with unnecessary ingredients such as sugar or agave nectar, plus cheap, inferior oils such as soy and canola. The best dressings are freshly made ones: Try a mix of olive oil and vinegar or lemon juice or tahini whisked with water, salt, and pepper.

PASTA

Pasta has never been considered a "health food," but varieties made from better ingredients can offer a healthier alternative to traditional pasta.

Look for varieties made from gluten-free grains or beans, such as quinoa, brown rice, chickpeas, and black beans. Check the ingredients list, though, as some alternative pastas still contain white, whole-wheat, or corn flours, which are less than optimal.

RASPBERRY FRUIT
SPREAD

APRICOT FRUIT SPREAD

MAYONNAISE

HORSERADISH

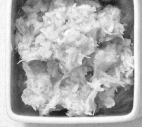

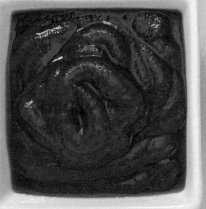

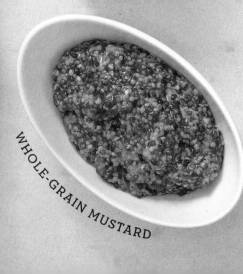

KETCHUP

WHOLE-GRAIN MUSTARD

KIMCHI

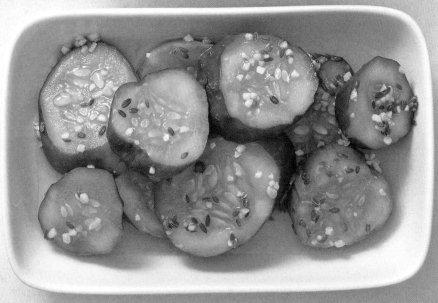

GARLIC DILL PICKLES

Watch out for whole-wheat pasta, which isn't much better than white pasta from a nutritional standpoint.

SOUPS

Look for soups in the refrigerator or freezer sections as these will be fresher and are less likely to contain preservatives, unnecessary additives, or excessive sugar.

Watch out for sugar. It doubles as a preservative, so many packaged foods contain high amounts of it to extend a product's shelf life.

SWEETENERS

Look for minimally processed or low glycemic sweeteners, such as date sugar, coconut sugar, raw honey, maple syrup, or stevia. Different sweeteners work better in different recipes, so it's a good idea to have a few on hand and use them accordingly.

Watch out for white or table sugar, which we know isn't healthy. However, there are also a number of other sweeteners with healthy halos around them that aren't much better than the white stuff. They include brown sugar, agave nectar, and artificial sweeteners.

Let's take a closer look at some of the better *natural* sweetener choices, but note, they should all still be used sparingly.

Organic Applesauce

Using applesauce instead of sugar in baking not only cuts calories substantially, it increases fiber and nutrients. Remember, apples are one of the most heavily pesticide-sprayed crops, so always choose organic.

Banana

Mashed banana can be used to sweeten baked goods or at least to reduce the amount of sugar in baked goods. It also makes a great smoothie base and when frozen and blended becomes a decadent "ice cream." By using a

whole food as a sweetener, you're getting the complete package of vitamins, minerals, and fiber as well, so the sugar is gentler on your body. (Note that it lends a banana-y taste to whatever you use it in.)

Dates & Date Sugar

You can use vitamin-, mineral-, and fiber-rich fresh or dried dates in many dessert recipes, or you can try date sugar, which consists of finely ground, dehydrated dates. If you like the taste of dates, this will definitely appeal to you. Date sugar can be used as a direct replacement for sugar and comes in granulated form. But it can clump, and it doesn't melt, making it an impractical substitution for certain baked goods and beverages. Dates are especially well suited to raw desserts.

Coconut Nectar & Coconut Sugar

Coconut palm sugar is lower on the glycemic index compared with white sugar—meaning it won't cause as large a spike in your blood sugar—and contains small amounts of vitamins, minerals, and amino acids. Because it's so versatile, tastes like regular sugar (not coconutty), and is low glycemic, it's one of the better direct replacements for white sugar. Note that it contains a decent amount of fructose, which has been linked to overeating and weight gain, but luckily, a little goes a long way. Many packages suggest you use it to replace sugar in a ratio of 1:1, but I typically use a lot less—usually half and sometimes even a third of that amount. It's available in both crystal and liquid forms.

Raw Honey (Preferably Local)

One of the oldest natural sweeteners, honey is sweeter than sugar. Depending on the plant source, honey can be dark and strong to light and mild in flavor. Raw honey contains small amounts of enzymes, minerals, and vitamins.

It may help increase immunity to common local allergens by introducing your body to small amounts of bee pollen. Raw honey looks whitish and opaque instead of yellowish and clear, like the traditional honey you'd find in a plastic squeeze bear. Most honey has been heated and processed, causing it to lose many of its healing properties and some nutritional value, so choose raw for the greatest benefits.

Maple Syrup

Maple syrup is made from boiled-down maple tree sap and is a source of both manganese and zinc. It adds a pleasant flavor to foods and is great for baking. Buy 100 percent pure maple syrup and not maple-flavored corn syrup. Choose Dark Color or Very Dark Color varieties, which are stronger in flavor and more nutritious than Golden or Amber Color varieties.

Monk Fruit Sweetener

This zero-calorie sweetener is made from an Asian fruit. It is sweeter than cane sugar but has no effect on blood sugar, making it the new darling of the health food world. Recently introduced to the U.S. market, monk fruit has been used for centuries in Eastern medicine to treat respiratory ailments and for general well-being. Now offered as a sweetener in crystal form, it seems to be one of the better sugar replacements on the market in terms of health and taste.

Stevia

Stevia is a leafy herb that's been used in South America for centuries. Stevia extract is *one hundred to three hundred* times sweeter than white sugar. It can be used in cooking, baking, and as a sugar substitute in most

❗ Expert Tip

Moderation is key. Though these alternative sweeteners are a better choice than processed white sugar, they should still be used in limited amounts. Don't go overboard!

beverages. Stevia doesn't affect blood sugar at all, which makes it a healthy choice.

Stevia is available in powder or liquid forms, but get the green or brown liquids or powders: The white and clear versions are highly refined. Avoid any stevia with the following ingredients: erythritol (which can cause digestive upset); natural flavors; and dextrose (which can be GMO).

Now that we know about some of the better natural sweetener alternatives, let's look at natural sweeteners that may not be as healthy as you think.

Agave Nectar

Agave nectar, or agave syrup, is a natural liquid sweetener made from the juice of the agave cactus. However, it is high in fructose and has been under much scrutiny due to how it's manufactured, which is similar to high fructose corn syrup. Research suggests that fructose affects the hormone leptin, which controls your appetite and satiety. Too much fructose may result in overeating and weight gain, so consume agave nectar in moderation or avoid it altogether.

Turbinado/Sugar in the Raw

Turbinado sugar, also known as demerara, is crystallized sugar made from sugar cane extract. It comes from the initial pressing of sugar cane, while white sugar is further refined. It's not very different from white sugar—just slightly less refined.

Oil

Like salt and pepper, oil is a staple when it comes to cooking. In recent years, the oil aisle has expanded to include more than a dozen varieties of oil: You can find oils made from all sorts of nuts, seeds, and fruit.

Oil is shunned in some health circles as it doesn't have a high nutritive value. It is relatively high in calories and is essentially pure fat, having had its fiber stripped away and taking vitamins and minerals with it. However, some healthy oils, such as olive oil, retain powerful phytonutrients linked to a reduced risk of certain cancers and heart disease. Still, even with healthy oils, moderation is key.

To reduce calories and boost nutrition, a great alternative to oils are the whole foods they come from. For instance, a dressing made from 1 tablespoon (15 ml) sesame oil would have about 120 calories and 0 minerals, while 1 tablespoon (15 g) tahini (sesame seed paste) contains only eighty-nine calories plus a small amount of calcium and iron.

Calorie and fat content aren't what makes certain oils unhealthy. What does, as you'll learn in the remainder of this section, is its source and the extraction and processing methods used to make it.

💰 Money-Saving Tip

Keep two types of olive oil on hand: extra-virgin olive oil for cold preparations such as dressings or drizzling over a dish after it's prepared, and virgin olive oil for cooking over low to medium-low heat. Although extra-virgin olive oil is the highest quality, best-tasting (and most expensive!) olive oil, it doesn't hold up well to heat, so use virgin olive oil for cooking. It's less expensive and has a higher smoke point!

Oil Buzzwords

There are a number of terms associated with oils, and olive oil even has its own unique set of legally defined terms. The first set of terms applies to all oils, and then a separate olive oil section follows.

EXPELLER PRESSED

This is a mechanical way of releasing oil in which the nut or seed is compressed at high pressure to force the oil out. The friction of the machine creates heat, which could be damaging to some oils, such as olive oil.

COLD PRESSED

Cold pressing is expeller pressing done under controlled cool temperatures to prevent oxidation or damage to delicate oils, such as olive oil. Cold pressing is the preferred extraction method because it releases the healthiest oil without inadvertently heating it and damaging the oil's integrity or nutrients.

REFINED

Refined oils are chemically extracted using a solvent—typically hexane, which is a by-product of gasoline refining. Besides being bathed in chemicals, refined oils undergo a number of processing steps. They're bleached, deodorized, and steam-cleaned before they make it into the bottle. These highly processed oils, commonly called "vegetable oils," are sold in plastic containers and should be avoided.

UNREFINED

Unrefined oil has not been treated with chemicals, bleach, or deodorizers after extraction.

Olive Oil Buzzwords

Unlike most oils, which are simply available as refined or unrefined, there's an entire vocabulary that accompanies olive oil. Become familiar with the following terms to make sure you're always getting the healthiest, highest-quality olive oil.

EXTRA-VIRGIN/FIRST COLD PRESSED

Extra-virgin is a term unique to olive oil and signifies the oil was cold pressed from the first pressing of olives, which results in the most pure, least acidic oil as well as the best-tasting oil. This is the highest-quality olive oil and is best used for drizzling instead of cooking. (You *can* cook with it at low temperatures—it's just more expensive.)

VIRGIN OLIVE OIL/COLD PRESSED

Virgin olive oil is also mechanically extracted, although its acidity is slightly higher. It's good for cooking over low to medium-low heat.

UNFILTERED OLIVE OIL

You may come across unfiltered olive oil with whitish sediment swirling around inside the bottle. It may be nutritionally superior to other olive oils, thanks to added antioxidants and nutrients in the sediment (the jury is still out on that, though). Use it only for dressings and cold preparations. Don't heat it: You'd just be degrading what you're paying a premium for!

OLIVE POMACE OIL

This is the oil obtained by treating olive pomace—the product remaining after the mechanical extraction of olive oil—with solvents or other chemical treatments. It's best avoided.

LIGHT OLIVE OIL

Light olive oil isn't lower in fat. It simply means that the oil is refined. Bottles labeled "100 percent pure olive oil" are the lowest quality olive oil and should be avoided.

> **❶ Expert Tip**
>
> **Top Four Tips for Selecting the Healthiest Oils**
>
> 1. Choose organic oils.
> 2. Chose cold-pressed or expeller-pressed oils.
> 3. Choose unrefined oils.
> 4. Choose oil that comes in glass or stainless steel containers.

Benefits of Oil

When used in moderation, unrefined oils can add flavor and a few health benefits.

SUPPORTS HEART HEALTH

Healthy oils, which are mechanically extracted from plant-based sources and contain monounsaturated and/or polyunsaturated fats, have been found to lower both cholesterol levels and the risk of heart disease. An example is first cold pressed olive oil.

ANTI-INFLAMMATORY

Healthy oils can help decrease inflammation in the body, which is beneficial for a variety of conditions as well as overall health.

Concerns About Oil

As mentioned earlier, not all oils are created equal. The highly processed oils are associated with more concerns than benefits. Here is what you should know:

REFINED OILS

As noted, refined oils are highly processed and treated with chemicals. Some of the chemicals may remain in the oil and harm your health. For example, the most common solvent, hexane, is neurotoxic. Examples of

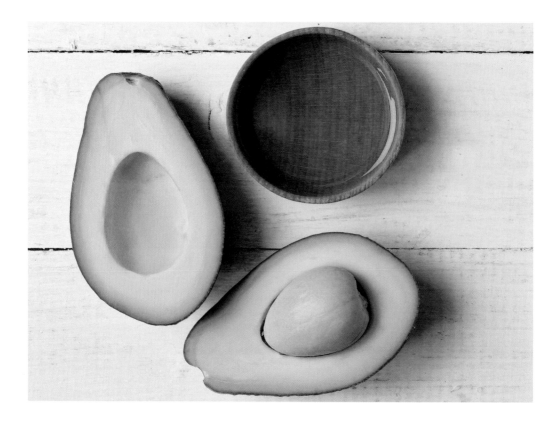

refined oils include vegetable oil, canola oil (unless it says expeller pressed), and corn oil.

PESTICIDES

Oils are highly concentrated, so pesticide and herbicide levels can be high even in small amounts. Choose organic oil to ensure you are consuming higher-quality raw ingredients and fewer chemicals.

OIL PACKAGING

The best storage containers for oil are made from glass or nonreactive metal, such as stainless steel. Tinted glass bottles are best, as they limit the amount of light that enters the bottle, keeping the oil fresher longer. Sometimes you'll find oil in plastic or metal containers that contain aluminum, copper,

or iron. Avoid these as they can leach toxic chemicals into the oil.

Healthiest Oils

The best oils are those that are unrefined and maintain the integrity of their delicate fats. The following top picks will suit any culinary need you may have:

AVOCADO OIL

Avocado oil has a high smoke point, making it excellent for high-heat cooking. Because it's mechanically extracted, it's superior to all other high-heat cooking oils, which are chemically extracted. Because avocado oil doesn't have a distinct flavor, it can be used for a variety of preparations. Always choose the unrefined version and look for it in a glass bottle.

COCONUT OIL

Coconut oil is a wonderful addition to your kitchen pantry. Besides its lightly tropical scent and flavor, it contains both antibacterial and antiviral properties and supports metabolism. If it's warm, the oil will look like a clear liquid, but if it's cool, it solidifies and turns white, which is typically how you see it at the grocery store. To liquefy it, simply place the jar in a hot water bath—or, put a spoonful right into a hot pan and it will melt instantly. Always choose the unrefined version and look for it in glass jars, not plastic.

Note: Some coconut oil producers now use the terms "virgin" or "extra virgin" to define their products. However, these are unregulated terms and may or may not be an indicator of actual quality.

OLIVE OIL

A staple of the Mediterranean diet, olive oil is rich in phytonutrients and antioxidants and provides anti-inflammatory benefits. It's excellent for drizzling on salads or incorporating into dressings, and you can cook with it, too, over low to medium-low heat. Choose extra-virgin olive oil for the most phytonutrients and health benefits when using as a dressing. Because extra-virgin olive oil has a low smoke point, use other oils, such as coconut or avocado, or even virgin olive oil (which has a higher smoke point), for medium-heat cooking.

Oil to Use Sparingly

Use the following oil only occasionally because of its high pro-inflammatory omega-6 fats.

SESAME OIL

Sesame oil has a light, delicate sesame flavor that features prominently in many Asian dishes. It's also often used in skincare and oral care routines in some Asian cultures, thanks to its antibacterial and antiviral properties. It's easy to find unrefined and expeller-pressed sesame oil, however, it is high in pro-inflammatory omega-6 fats, which should be avoided in large amounts.

You can offset this by using it sparingly or occasionally or in dishes that contain large amounts of anti-inflammatory omega-3s, including salmon, sardines, soy, Brussels sprouts, or cauliflower. Though the other oils listed are better options for cooking, if you do

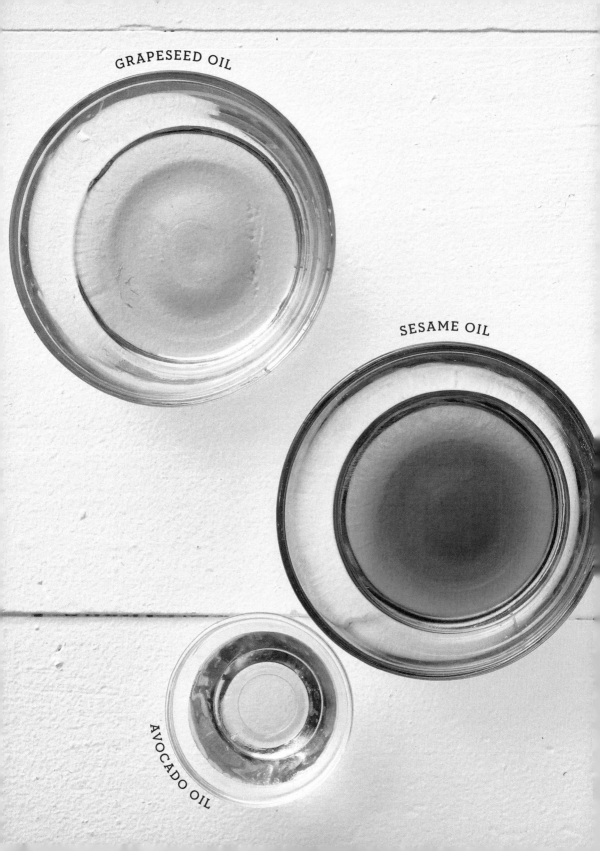

GRAPESEED OIL

SESAME OIL

AVOCADO OIL

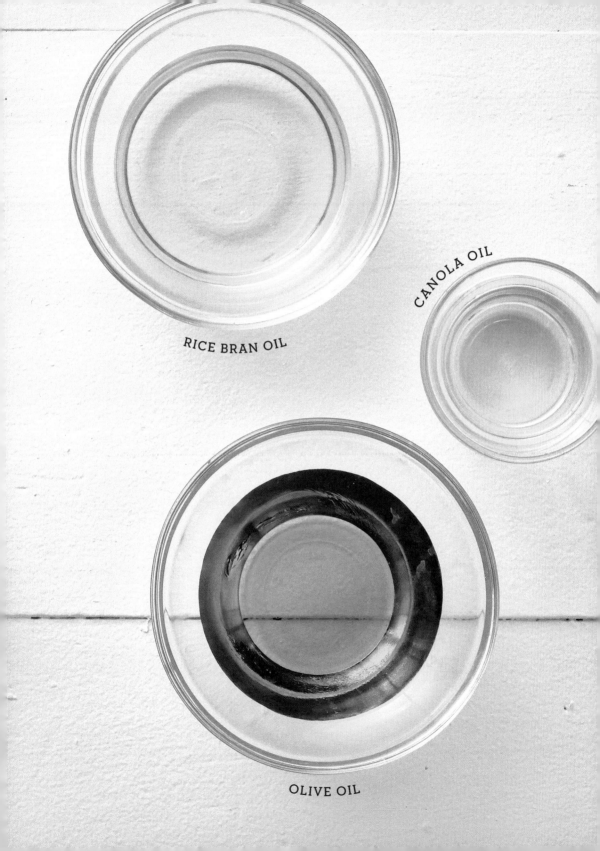

RICE BRAN OIL

CANOLA OIL

OLIVE OIL

use sesame oil that way, limit its use to low to medium heat. Or, reserve it for your skin and oral care routines.

The Least Healthy Oils

The following oils have been refined and chemically extracted. If a bottle is not labeled "expeller pressed" or "cold pressed," assume it was chemically extracted.

You can spot them easily: They're pale in color, highly translucent, neutral tasting, and usually sold in plastic containers (although sometimes you'll find them in glass or metal bottles). On the bottle, look for the word "refined" and/or the absence of the words "cold pressed" or "expeller pressed."

Oils are refined so they can withstand higher cooking temperatures. However, the refining process exposes the oil to heat and chemicals that diminish its quality and health value. Plus, the most common refined oils, such as canola, corn, and soy, are also typically GMO, and many are high in pro-inflammatory omega-6 fatty acids.

For optimum health, consider limiting or avoiding the following oils, both for cooking and in packaged products.

CANOLA OIL

Due to its omega-3 content, canola oil is often mistakenly touted as "healthy." But with the way rapeseed—the seed canola oil is made from—is grown and processed, it's anything but good for you. More than 90 percent of canola oil is genetically modified, and all of it is chemically extracted, which involves high temperatures and chemicals of questionable safety. Plus, because omega-3 fatty acids become rancid and foul smelling at high temperatures—and when exposed to oxygen, as they are during processing—the oil is then deodorized by converting a large amount of the omega-3s into trans fat. This may not turn up on the nutrition label, but it certainly makes it into the bottle. Research at the University of Florida, Gainesville, found trans fats levels as high as 4.6 percent in commercial canola oil.

CORN OIL

Corn oil has been dubbed "the unhealthiest oil" for a number of reasons. It is chemically extracted, GMO, and high in pro-inflammatory omega-6 fatty acids.

GRAPESEED OIL

Grapeseed oil is a byproduct of the wine industry. It's made from the seeds of pressed grapes that would traditionally be discarded. The oil, which is extremely high in pro-inflammatory omega-6 fats, is released through chemical extraction methods.

PEANUT OIL

Peanut oil is commonly used in Asian dishes, and it's the oil of choice for deep-fryers (and deep-fried foods are not healthy). Like the other oils on this list, it too is high in pro-inflammatory omega-6 fats.

RICE BRAN OIL

Rice bran oil is also chemically extracted and high in pro-inflammatory omega-6 fatty acids.

SAFFLOWER OIL

Like other refined oils, safflower oil has a neutral flavor and is often used in high-heat cooking. Although it's often expeller pressed, it's generally refined afterward, making most brands of safflower oil poor choices. Additionally, it's high in pro-inflammatory omega-6 fatty acids.

If you do find safflower oil that's both expeller pressed and unrefined—which is

Oil Smoke Points

Every oil has a smoke point—a temperature at which it literally starts to smoke. When this happens, the fat in the oil starts to break down, releasing free radicals and a substance called acrolein, the chemical that gives burnt foods their acrid flavor and aroma. Free radicals are damaging to the body on many levels and should be avoided. Therefore, the oil you use should depend on the heat level at which you're cooking. However, if you leave a pan of oil over the heat for too long and it starts to smoke, carefully dispose of the oil and start over.

Following are the top oil choices for everyday cooking:

- For dressings or cold preparations: extra-virgin olive oil (bonus points for unfiltered)

- In place of butter: avocado oil, coconut oil, or olive oil, depending on the dish

- Low to medium heat: virgin olive oil or unrefined coconut oil

- For high-heat cooking: avocado oil

food, and most people use it as a source of highly anti-inflammatory omega-3s. However, you'll notice that flax oil is always sold in the refrigerator section because it goes rancid very quickly. Rancid oils are toxic to the body and can be carcinogenic, inflammatory, and promote advanced aging. If you're looking for omega-3s, freshly milled flaxseed is a better choice than the oil. If you use the oil, *never cook with it*. And, if it tastes off, it's probably gone bad and should be thrown out.

PANTRY STAPLES

uncommon, though it does exist—remember there are healthier options. Safflower oil is low in omega-3s and high in omega-6s.

SOYBEAN OIL
Soybean oil is chemically extracted and typically, GMO.

VEGETABLE OIL
Vegetable oil is usually made from soybean oil or a blend of unhealthy oils, including canola and sunflower, so it's typically GMO and pro-inflammatory.

FLAXSEED OIL (HEALTHY HALO!)
Flax oil has a nutty flavor, but it's not typically consumed for its taste. It's touted as a health

CHAPTER 14

FROZEN FOODS

In some respects, we've come a long way from the original frozen TV dinners. There are more organic, gluten-free, non-GMO food options in the supermarket's freezer aisle than ever before. While fresh food is typically the better choice, incorporating certain frozen foods into your diet can offer you convenience without having to sacrifice health. As with the rest of the grocery store, though, choose whole foods (such as frozen vegetables) over more highly processed foods (such as an enchilada).

Excellent frozen food choices include vegetables, fruit, legumes, and grains, all of which make eating real food convenient and affordable. You do, however, have to be a bit more careful when it comes to prepared meals and desserts. There are, indeed, healthier options in these categories, but, of course, there are still some questionable "foods" lingering in the freezer section. As always, reading the ingredients list will help you determine a product's quality before you purchase (and eat) it.

Tips for Selecting the Healthiest Frozen Foods

Look for mainly whole ingredients: frozen vegetables, fruit, and precooked grains and beans. For premade meals, stick with high-quality veggie burgers or vegetable-based entrées with simple, wholesome ingredients and no additives. And many frozen meals contain excess sodium, so look for those labeled low- or no-sodium.

On the flip side, *watch out for* and avoid frozen foods with partially hydrogenated oils, added sugars, excessive sodium (more than 600 milligrams per serving), or ingredients you wouldn't stock in your own kitchen. Don't be fooled by "diet" dinners: These are not nearly as healthy as they sound. Always read the ingredients list, and if products are loaded with unfamiliar, synthetic ingredients instead of real foods, steer clear. Also, if the calorie count is too low—around 200 calories—the meal probably won't fill you up or offer the nutrients or energy you need, which may just lead to more snacking later on. A meal should be between 350 and 500 calories.

Top Freezer Aisle Picks

Stocking your freezer will cut down food prep time—and can even save a little money. Follow this advice to select the healthiest options for you and your family.

FROZEN FRUIT & VEGETABLES

Frozen fruits and vegetables make an excellent nutritional—and economical—choice. Though quite a bit less expensive than fresh produce, they're typically just as nutritious, if not more so. That's because they're picked

Top Five Frozen Foods to Stock Up On

1. Frozen fruits and vegetables
2. Frozen beans
3. Frozen precooked grains
4. Veggie burgers with real, whole ingredients
5. Gluten-free, preservative-free breads or baked goods

Top Five Frozen Foods to Avoid

1. Frozen dinners
2. Low-calorie "diet" dinners
3. Frozen french fries or sweet potato fries
4. Frozen chicken nuggets
5. Ice cream

when ripe and the most nutrient dense and then immediately flash-frozen, helping retain those nutrients. The only exceptions to this are broccoli and carrots, which don't retain their nutrients well when frozen. Add frozen fruit to smoothies; turn it into jams; or use in desserts. Steam—never boil—frozen vegetables to maintain maximum nutrition.

FROZEN PRECOOKED RICE & GRAINS

You can now find precooked, frozen rice and grains that require only a few minutes to reheat instead of the better part of half an hour to cook from scratch. This is good in a pinch; however, for more flavor and about the same convenience, you can also make a larger batch of rice or grains early in the week and refrigerate and reheat as needed. Or, invest in a pressure cooker to cook rice (and dried beans) fast.

FROZEN PRECOOKED BEANS

Beans take a long time to cook from scratch, and canned varieties aren't ideal due to concerns over chemicals in the can's lining. Happily, you can now find precooked frozen beans, which can be easily defrosted or reheated. If you use beans often and want to save money, consider making large batches of beans in a pressure cooker and freezing them yourself.

FROZEN BREAD & TORTILLAS

You'll find a wide variety of frozen breads and tortillas made without preservatives that are superior in quality to the types with nearly immortal shelf lives in the dry goods aisle. Keep them frozen at home—or, if you plan to eat the whole loaf in a week or less, in the refrigerator. Look for gluten-free, sprouted, or sourdough varieties. For tortillas, try brown rice or sprouted corn options.

Best Freezer Section Swaps

Though the temptation exists to fill your grocery cart with frozen convenience foods and premade meals, the health benefits are huge if you make a few simple substitutions instead. Get ready to swap!

SWAP FROZEN DINNERS FOR ONE-POT MEALS

Although convenient, frozen dinners are nutritionally subpar and often contain ingredients that detract from your health, such as low-quality oils, fillers, sugar, and preservatives.

Instead, for quick weeknight meals, try a healthy (real food) veggie burger—or buy a variety of frozen whole foods, such as vegetables, legumes, or grains, and then throw together a quick stir-fry or veggie curry with just a few extra ingredients.

SWAP FROZEN "DIET" DINNERS FOR 350- TO 500-CALORIE MEALS

If you've read this far, you know that calorie count is not the best indicator of a product's health value. For instance, two hundred calories of highly processed ravioli probably won't fill you up, and it most definitely won't bring you closer to meeting your nutrient needs. When you eat these low-calorie, nutritionally bankrupt foods, you're likely to be hungry again soon and may end up overeating. Plus, they often contain a variety of fillers, preservatives, and other artificial ingredients.

Instead, cook a simple meal using some quinoa and steaming a bag of frozen vegetables. Be generous with spices to add flavor, and dinner will be ready in ten minutes!

SWAP FROZEN PIZZA FOR HOMEMADE

Though not a health food, if the desire for pizza strikes, there are a few gluten-free crust and nondairy-cheese options that can minimize the risk of bloating and gut inflammation for the gluten- and dairy-intolerant.

Homemade pizza is a quick, healthier option. Here's a simple recipe: Bake a (frozen) brown rice tortilla at 400°F (200°C, or gas mark 6) for about seven to ten minutes until crisp before adding your choice of toppings. Return the tortilla to the oven for another five to ten minutes.

Or, try your hand at making the popular cauliflower crust pizzas—or buy a dry gluten-free pizza crust mix. No matter what you use as your base, be sure to pile on the sauce and veggies.

SWAP FROZEN VEGGIE BURGERS FOR REAL-FOOD VEGGIE BURGERS

Not only do most veggie burgers taste terrible but they are highly processed and loaded with undesirable ingredients, such as soy protein, whey, dairy, fillers, chemicals, preservatives, and excessive sodium.

Instead, choose a clean veggie burger made solely from beans, quinoa, vegetables, and/or nuts. (Of course, the only way you'll know what's inside is to read the ingredients list!) Skip the bun, top it with avocado, and serve with a big side salad or baked sweet potato wedges.

SWAP FROZEN FRENCH FRIES FOR HOMEMADE SWEET POTATO WEDGES

Although baked sweet potato fries are, indeed, a better choice than regular potato fries, the frozen versions often contain undesirable ingredients such as inferior oils, sugar, and GMO cornstarch that are best avoided. What's more, even though you're baking the fries, they were almost certainly pre-fried and drenched in oil.

Easily make your own by cutting sweet potatoes into shoestrings or wedges. Then coat with olive oil and your favorite spices. Roast at 450°F (230°C, or gas mark 8) for twenty minutes or so. It doesn't take much longer than opening a bag of frozen fries!

SWAP FROZEN CHICKEN NUGGETS FOR HOMEMADE NUGGETS

Even when labeled "all natural" and "gluten-free," frozen chicken nuggets aren't usually a good choice. They often contain a variety of preservatives, artificial fillers, trans fat, and excess sodium—plus, they're pre-fried. (Fried is never good.)

Make your own nuggets so you can choose the highest-quality organic meat and type of breading while also avoiding any unnecessary fillers. Or, skip the nuggets and replace them with a grilled or baked chicken dish instead.

If it's the nugget look and feel you're after, though, look for mini frozen veggie burger bites in health food stores. They look like chicken nuggets, but come with added fiber and nutrients.

SWAP FROZEN FISH FILLETS FOR FROZEN WILD FISH

Skip the breaded and fried fish fillets, which, like chicken nuggets, are pre-fried and probably contain a variety of fillers and preservatives, plus excess sodium.

Heading to the fishmonger isn't a bad idea, but opting for frozen fillets is more economical and just as nutritious. Approximately 70 percent or more of fish—and all wild-caught fish—sold at fish markets has been frozen, according ot the National Fisheries Institute. Frozen fish can last a few months, depending on the type of fish and the packaging.

SWAP REGULAR ICE CREAM FOR COCONUT- OR NUT-BASED ICE CREAM

Ice cream is by no means a health food, but when that craving strikes, know there are better options than traditional cream-based, artificially flavored, sugar-laden products. In light of the health concerns linked to dairy outlined in chapter 11, look for nondairy ice creams made from coconut or nuts. Both produce creamy, decadent treats, so you won't feel like you're missing a thing. If you find one sweetened with natural sweeteners—dates, honey, coconut sugar, or maple syrup—that's an even better choice.

CHAPTER 15

SNACKS & SWEETS

Americans have become serial snackers. The latest government statistics show that, as of 2010, more than 90 percent of the population consumes at least one snack a day. That's up from 59 percent in 1978. Currently, the majority of Americans—56 percent—snack three or more times a day, up from 10 percent in the late 1970s.

Americans first shifted from three square meals a day about 100 years ago at fairs and circuses where popcorn, peanuts, and candied apples were for sale. Then snacking was tied to fun and entertainment. Once considered an indulgence, snacking has now become the norm.

There is no consensus on whether it's better to eat three meals or multiple smaller snacks throughout the day. However, it's clear that most typical snack foods are best avoided, even in small portions. Don't be fooled by low calorie counts: Common snack foods are nutritionally bankrupt. Devoid of nutrients and fiber, they won't satisfy for long and increase your chances of overeating your daily calories. Plus, they tend to be high in salt, sugar, processed oils, chemical ingredients, artificial flavors, and preservatives.

The best snacks are, naturally, whole foods. Think crisp crudités with guacamole, tapenade, or hummus; raw or sprouted nuts and seeds; or fresh fruit. It's much harder to overeat these types of foods because they contain fiber to fill you and nutrients your body needs. Studies have shown, for example, that when people snack on raw nuts, they usually eat fewer calories at later meals—but when people snack on empty-calorie foods, such as low-calorie cookies, they eat the same amount of calories as usual at later meals. The paradox is that at the end of the day, the "low-calorie" snacker ends up eating more calories than the real-food snacker.

As people get wise to the pitfalls of snack foods, a wave of food companies has stepped in to offer healthier snack options that are still convenient. From seasoned and sprouted nuts to seaweed to cookies made solely from nuts and fruit, you now have access to a wide range of delicious, nutritious, snackable options. Here I outline the top picks and swaps for a variety of packaged snacks and sweets to fulfill your snacking urge.

Savory Snack Swaps

Most savory snacks are fried and contain excessive amounts of sodium. Instead, look for versions that are baked, low in salt (or, even better, seasoned with pink Himalayan or Celtic salt), and use healthier oils, such as coconut, olive, or avocado.

As we did with frozen foods, to ensure you choose the healthiest options, get ready, again, to swap traditional processed snacks for healthier options!

SWAP TRADITIONAL CORN OR POTATO CHIPS FOR ORGANIC VEGGIE CHIPS

Chips are easy to overeat as the marriage of salt, fat, and crunch makes them nearly irresistible. Most are fried and made from corn—likely GMO—plus inferior, inflammatory oils. Certain varieties also contain artificial colors, flavors, and preservatives.

Instead choose from the ever-growing assortment of better options: organic corn, kale, sweet potato, and other veggie chips made with healthier oils and/or baked instead of fried. And many are made with organic and non-GMO vegetables, healthier oils, such as coconut or olive oil, and Himalayan or Celtic salt. Although they'll never be on a nutritional par with unprocessed foods, these are a smarter option than the conventional choices.

SWAP TRADITIONAL FLOUR-BASED CRACKERS FOR GLUTEN-FREE WHOLE-GRAIN OR NUT & SEED CRACKERS

Most crackers are made from wheat or white flour and do little to satisfy your hunger—or your nutritional needs.

When you want something crunchy, choose crackers made from gluten-free whole grains instead of whole-grain flour. These offer superior nutrition and increased satiety, plus more stable blood sugar levels. You can also find crackers made from nuts and seeds—often in the raw foods aisle at a health food store.

SWAP ROASTED, SALTED NUTS & SEEDS FOR RAW OR SPROUTED VERSIONS

Skip the heavy roasted nuts, which contain excessive amounts of inferior oils and sodium. Instead, choose raw or soaked and sprouted nuts and seeds. If it's flavor you're after, a number of brands offer seasoned sprouted nuts, flavored with a variety of herbs and spices.

SWAP MICROWAVE POPCORN & CONVENTIONAL PRE-POPPED POPCORN FOR ORGANIC

Microwave popcorn typically contains deadly trans fats in the form of partially hydrogenated oils. And conventional corn, we know, is typically GMO and associated with a range of possible health concerns.

Always choose organic or non-GMO verified popcorn to avoid GMOs and select pre-popped or whole kernels instead of microwave versions to avoid any unnecessary additives, such as trans fats, artificial flavors, and excessive sodium. These days, there are a few brands that offer organic pre-popped popcorn made with healthier oils, such as olive or coconut, and that are even seasoned with pink Himalayan or Celtic salt.

SWAP PROTEIN & MEAL BARS FOR FRUIT & NUT BARS

Most protein and meal bars are loaded with sugar and empty, or even harmful, ingredients such as soy protein isolate and whey protein. Whey protein is a waste by-product of the dairy industry, and although it is high in protein, it's still dairy based, so it has the same associated concerns and isn't the best protein source. Soy protein isolate is a controversial, highly processed form of soy, devoid of all of its natural vitamins, minerals, fiber, healthy fats, and carbs.

Although they can be devoured in just a few bites, lower-quality (yet popular) bars often contain a laundry list of ingredients, including artificial flavors, vitamins, or chemicals.

Choose bars that get their protein from plant-based sources, such as nuts, seeds, or peas. The ingredients list for a bar should generally contain fruit (usually dates) and nuts, seeds, and/or grains. Beyond protein, these types of bars also offer a variety of

DRIED COCONUT

DRIED FIGS

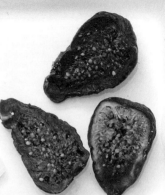

RAW
COCOA AND COCONUT
BITES

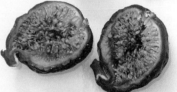

SPROUTED
CARROT
COOKIES

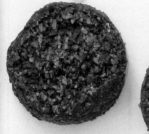

RAW
LEMON COCONUT
BITES

**DARK CHOCOLATE
WITH ALMONDS**

DATE ROLLS

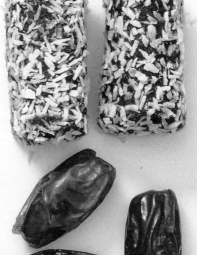

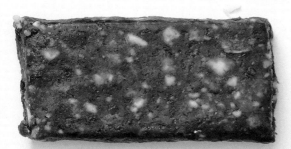

FRUIT & NUT BARS

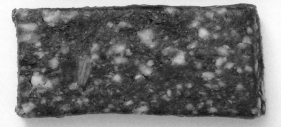

DRIED DATES

natural vitamins and minerals. And, as far as sweeteners go, dates are healthier than added sugar—even the brown rice syrup, agave nectar, or other sugar syrups typically used in bars. Because the whole fruit is used, you get added fiber and nutrients.

SWAP REGULAR PRETZELS FOR GLUTEN-FREE WHOLE-GRAIN PRETZELS

Pretzels, typically made with little more than flour, water, and salt, are an empty-calorie food. Any nutrients they contain have been added synthetically in the form of enriched flour. Because they're refined and low in fiber and protein, they won't fill you up for long.

If you crave pretzels, look for gluten-free whole-grain versions with clean ingredients. (Remember, just because it's gluten-free doesn't mean it's automatically a healthy choice!) Avoid versions with conventional corn-based ingredients (likely GMO) or ingredients that are overly chemical based.

Instead opt for pretzels made from gluten-free whole grains or nuts and seeds, such as brown rice, quinoa, or millet. If you're just looking for crunch, nuts and seeds are a healthier, whole food option. If you need a salt fix, try seaweed snacks.

SWAP SALTY SNACKS FOR ROASTED SEAWEED

What do you do when you crave something salty? Chips? Pretzels? The most common options are often fried or contain empty calories and excessive sodium—and don't support good health (or our waistlines!) However, rich in minerals and iodine, seaweed makes a nutritious, yet salty alternative. And because the snack-size versions have just five calories, this is one snack you can double—or triple!—up on. They're not very filling, but they're a fun, tasty way to get your iodine. For a more filling snack, buy the larger sheets of roasted seaweed or nori and roll sliced avocado or vegetables in them to make sushi-style wraps.

Sweets Swaps

Sugar might not be great for your health, but life without sweets would not be any fun. Satisfy your sweet tooth with desserts made with gentler natural sugars, such as fruit or coconut sugar. Here are some ideas for healthier versions of your favorite sweets.

SWAP CANDY FOR DARK CHOCOLATE OR DATE ROLLS

With all of its sugar, artificial colors, and ingredients, you could never mistake candy for health food. While there's no good direct replacement for candy, you can wean yourself off the sweet stuff by switching to dark chocolate or date rolls.

Dark chocolate has drastically less added sugar, and its slight bitterness should slow you down so you don't overeat. Look for bars that are 72 percent or, ideally, 85 percent cacao or even higher.

Date rolls—date paste rolled in coconut—are another good option. They're super-sweet, but still have natural fiber and nutrients.

SWAP FRUIT YOGURT FOR CHIA PUDDING

Fruit yogurt can seem like a quick and convenient snack, but the fruit-flavored varieties are typically loaded with added sugar.

Chia pudding is high in fiber and protein, making it an energizing snack that'll keep you going for hours. It's usually made with coconut or almond milk instead of dairy and sometimes sweetened with fruit or coconut sugar.

SWAP MILK CHOCOLATE FOR DARK CHOCOLATE

Chocolate is sometimes demonized as the cause of breakouts and weight gain, but the

Making the Switch to Dark Chocolate

If you're new to dark chocolate and your taste buds are still used to the sugary stuff, start with 60 percent dark chocolate. Take a week or two to get used to it and then switch to 70 percent. After you get used to that, move up to 85 percent and stay put. Chocolate that's 99 percent cacao is super-bitter: It's only for the most hard-core chocophiles!

cacao—or cocoa—isn't to blame: The added sugar and dairy are likely the real culprits. Some milk chocolate may also contain artificial flavors and even colors. Versions that list sugar as the first ingredient should really be called "sugar bars" as they actually contain more sugar than cocoa!

Dark chocolate, on the other hand, is often praised for its health benefits. It contains a higher percentage of cacao, which is loaded with minerals and antioxidants. Look for brands with a cocoa content of at least 72 percent or, ideally, 85 percent or above—an indicator of more antioxidants and less sugar. Find one without dairy ingredients (milk, milk powder, etc.) and with a gentle natural sweetener, such as coconut sugar, date sugar, maple syrup, or stevia.

SWAP DRIED FRUIT FOR DRIED COCONUT

There are worse things to snack on than dried fruit, but because the fruit's water content has been removed, you can end up ingesting quite a bit more—and, therefore, more sugar—than you normally would if eating whole fruit.

Some dried fruit—particularly tart fruit, such as cherries and cranberries—usually have added sugar. Nonorganic dried fruit typically contains sulfites, which are used as preservatives; some people are sensitive to them.

Tropical-tasting dried coconut chips, chunks, or slices make for a delightful, satisfying snack that's naturally low in sugar. Because they're not super sweet and are loaded with healthy fats, fiber, and protein, you can't (and won't even want to!) eat the whole bag. If you're going to eat dried fruit, the best choices include the following:

Dates: Dates taste sinfully sweet, but offer a surprising variety of health benefits. They contain at least fifteen minerals, including selenium, an element that supports healthy immune function. They also contain a variety of powerful antioxidants, such as quercetin, which may help protect against cardiovascular disease. What's more, a study published in *Nutrition Journal* found that dates don't significantly spike blood glucose.

Figs: Fresh figs are a delicacy available only for a few short months each year, but dried figs are available year-round. They're a good source of fiber as well as potassium and calcium, which support bone health.

Goji berries: This "superfood" is extremely high in vitamin A, an essential nutrient for clear skin, and a variety of antioxidants. These berries contain more than twenty trace minerals.

SWAP COOKIES FOR DATE ROLLS

Traditional cookies don't offer much in the way of nutrition because they're usually little more than flour and sugar.

If it must be a cookie, look for gluten-free ones sweetened with a low glycemic sweeter such as coconut sugar—or even fruit, such as dates. As always, check the ingredients and choose brands with the simplest ingredients.

For healthier options, your best bet is to visit the raw or vegan section of the grocery store, where you can find "cookies" made from nothing but dates, sesame, and coconut.

But if you want something sweet that isn't necessarily a cookie, try date rolls— date paste rolled in coconut, nuts, or seeds. They're a great alternative to your afternoon cookie habit!

Date rolls are available in the bulk section (or packaged in the produce section), but it's easy to make your own. Blend dates in a bullet blender with shredded coconut to form a paste. Then roll the paste into logs and coat them with additional shredded coconut.

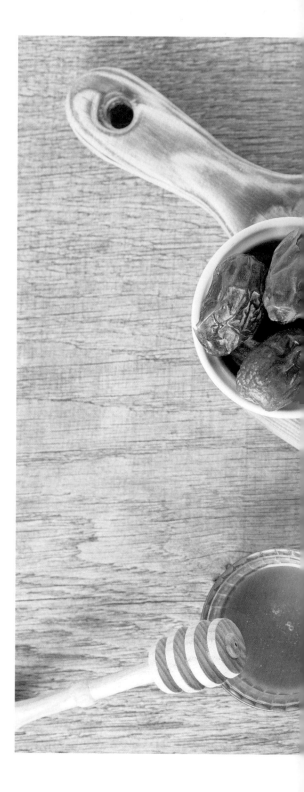

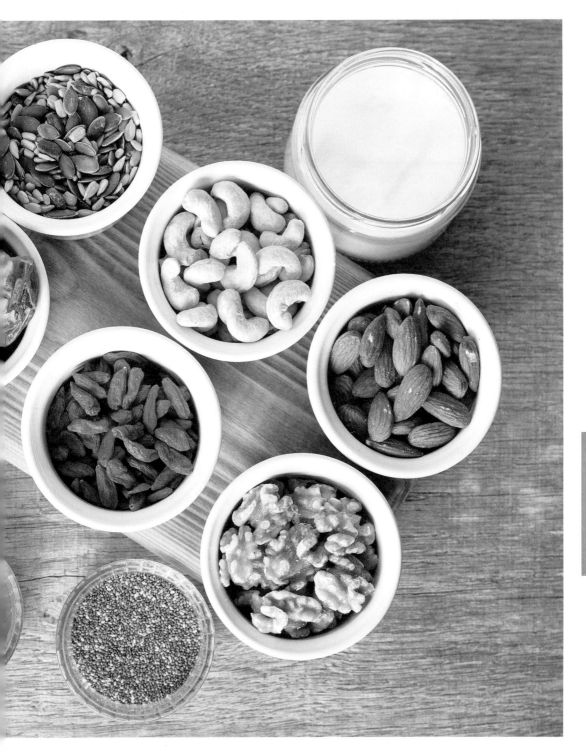

CHAPTER 16

BEVERAGES

The ever-expanding beverage aisle is packed with all sorts of juices, iced teas, sodas, and functional elixirs. There has been plenty of growth in the coffee and tea aisle, too, where it's easy to be overwhelmed by the number of choices.

Beverages are often a sneaky place for sugar or other unnecessary additives to hide: So, as with other packaged foods, bypass the front label and head straight to the ingredients list. But even that's not always enough. For example, when it comes to juice, you'll also want to know how it was processed, as processing methods substantially change its health value.

It goes without saying that water is the healthiest beverage of all. But what if you're craving something sweet and bubbly or a hot cuppa joe? This chapter shows you how to make the healthiest choices.

Best Beverage Choices

Following are the best beverage choices to help keep you hydrated and healthy.

WATER

When you consider the amount of water you should drink each day for optimal health, buying a high-quality water filter for your drinking water is much more economical than buying bottles of it. What's more, it's also healthier because the hormone-disrupting chemicals used to make plastic bottles can leach into the water. A study published in *PLOS ONE* found that a single bottle of water could contain more than twenty-four thousand chemicals, two classes of which—maleates and fumarates—are known endocrine disruptors.

If you need more convincing that filtered tap is better than bottled, it's estimated that about 25 percent of bottled water is bottled tap water! If it's packaged as "purified" or "drinking water," chances are it came from a municipal water supply. Aquafina and Dasani, the two most popular brands of bottled water, are from municipal supplies.

As much of our public tap water is chlorinated and fluoridated, select a filter that removes both of these chemicals. Once you switch to filtered tap water, you'll not only avoid endocrine-disrupting chemicals from plastic bottles, you'll also save thousands of bottles from ending up in landfills during your lifetime.

Look for glass-bottled water from a spring or natural source—or, even better, invest in a high-quality water filter and filter your tap water.

Watch out for plastic-bottled water, especially if it's labeled as purified or drinking water: It's nothing more than tap water.

COCONUT WATER

Fresh coconut water has such a unique taste—deliciously sweet and nutty. When tapped straight from a young coconut, it is rich in nutrients and electrolytes, including potassium, magnesium, and manganese. It's sometimes called "nature's sports drink" because it's certainly a healthier source of electrolytes than the artificially colored and flavored sugary sports drinks on the market. Some grocery stores sell fresh young coconuts. You can chop the top off—and stick a straw right inside!—to reach the delicious water. This is your best option.

Shelf-stable or bottled coconut waters, on the other hand, generally have added ingredients and are so highly processed they taste nothing like the original. There are better tasting and more nutritious options.

An in-between option, which is the next best thing to a fresh coconut, is the bottled coconut waters found in the refrigerator or freezer sections. These are typically unpasteurized, resulting in better flavor and nutrient maintenance. They should have only one ingredient—coconut water.

Look for whole coconuts or frozen or refrigerated bottled coconut waters without any added ingredients. Ideally, choose unpasteurized versions for best flavor.

Watch out for boxed coconut waters and coconut waters with added ingredients.

JUICE

Fresh-pressed juice made at home or in a health food store can be a healthy drink, but the versions in grocery stores have been processed nearly to the point of nutrient extinction. They don't retain the life-giving, glow-inducing benefits as fresh juice and typically aren't much more than liquid sugar. Plus, as discussed previously, certain companies use flavor packs to make their orange juice taste exactly the same—all year long, anywhere in the world—but they don't list the additional ingredients in the ingredients list.

Although there are a variety of newer, "cleaner" brands on the market, remember the processing that allows the juice—a highly perishable product—to sit on shelves for weeks at a time reduces its nutrient value, making it a waste of calories. Besides, packaged juice never tastes as good as the fresh version!

So, if you're in the mood for juice, make your own or head to a juice bar and buy it fresh. Ideally, choose one that's vegetable based or that has a non-sweet fruit as its base—think cucumber or lemon—to limit the amount of sugar.

BEVERAGES

Look for freshly made unpasteurized juices at health food stores or juice bars. Cold-pressed juice retains the most nutrients. Green or vegetable juices are best. There is a risk of bacterial contamination associated with consuming unpasteurized products—for example, when fruit or veggies used in the juice weren't washed properly before juicing and contained bacteria. Always buy juice from a reputable source with high-quality standards.

Watch out for juices that are shelf stable (that is, not sold in the refrigerated section), pasteurized juices, or those with a shelf life longer than three days.

KOMBUCHA

Kombucha is a health food store favorite and has quickly eaten up shelf space in the refrigerated beverage section. This traditional Asian beverage is a type of fermented tea that's slightly effervescent and enjoyed cold. High-quality brands are unsweetened or use just a touch of fruit or vegetable juice for flavor. It's claimed that kombucha has a wide variety of health benefits, although there isn't yet much research to prove that. It can be a healthier alternative to more commonly consumed, overly sweetened beverages.

Look for kombucha in glass bottles, without any added sugar—a little bit of fruit juice is okay, though.

Watch out for kombucha with added sugar.

CHIA DRINKS

Functional drinks are elbowing their way into the beverage aisle and that includes chia drinks. As explained in chapter 7, chia is a nutritional powerhouse, providing anti-inflammatory omega-3s, protein, and fiber. It's extremely filling and aids digestion.

Look for chia drinks made with fruit juice or sweetened with stevia. While pasteurized juices—including most chia drinks—are not

ideal, this is one of the better choices if you want something other than water.

Watch out for chia drinks with added sugar.

APPLE CIDER VINEGAR DRINKS

Apple cider vinegar is a health food store staple, and though you can take a shot of it "neat" to aid digestion or overall health, there are diluted apple cider vinegar beverages sweetened with stevia or honey on the market. If you want something other than water that still supports your health, try one of these.

Look for apple cider vinegar drinks sweetened with honey or stevia in glass bottles.

Watch out for any with added sugar.

BEET KVASS

As probiotics become more popular, more and more fermented drinks (which contain natural probiotics) are hitting the market. Kvass is a traditionally fermented beverage that has a similar taste to beer. It's often made from sourdough bread. However, the ones that pop up in health food stores are more likely to be made from nutrient-rich beets.

Look for unsweetened versions or those that use a gentler sweetener, such as stevia, and check the ingredients before choosing.

Watch out for any with added sugar or other additives.

❗ Expert Tip

If you're in the mood for a freshly squeezed fruit juice but don't want the blood sugar spike, throw a tablespoon (13 g) or so of chia seeds into your juice and let it sit for five to ten minutes before drinking. The chia seeds will be suspended in the juice, becoming virtually undetectable when you sip it—but their fiber and protein will help minimize the blood sugar spike.

Beverage Swaps

Get ready to do some swapping—you know the drill by now. Replace those not-so-good-for-you beverages with ones that will do your body some good, without feeling deprived.

SWAP SODA. PERIOD.

Let's get one thing straight: Soda, unfortunately, will never be considered "healthy." (Especially not diet soda! The artificial sweeteners make it even worse than the sweetened version.) All soda, whether regular or diet, is either liquid sugar or liquid chemicals, and your body doesn't ever need them—not even on special occasions.

A University of Texas study found that drinking one to two cans of diet soda daily increases your risk of obesity by 54.5 percent, compared to 32.8 percent for people who drink the same amount of regular soda. (So much for losing weight with diet drinks.) And a study by the University of Miami's Miller School of Medicine found that regular consumption of diet cola increases your risk of a cardiac event by 61 percent. Finally, artificial sweeteners are believed to be neurotoxins, meaning they can excite your brain cells to the point of cell death. So . . .

If you like the taste and mouthfeel of bubbles, swap regular and diet soda for seltzer water, kombucha, or an alternative soda sweetened with stevia. If you're drinking an alternative soda, think of it as a transition beverage to help wean your taste buds off the sugar and bubbles, rather than as a permanent replacement.

SWAP BOTTLED ICED TEA FOR HOMEMADE

A hot cup of freshly brewed tea is, indeed, loaded with antioxidants and other benefits, but the nutrition is a bit different when it comes to bottled iced tea. Manufacturers typically add a lot of sugar to iced teas, negating any health benefits. Some use high fructose corn syrups and added flavors and preservatives, too. Drinking sugar is particularly bad for your waistline, so don't mistake bottled iced teas for a healthy beverage.

Better options include unsweetened options or those sweetened with a (slightly) healthier sweetener, such as honey. But these are few and far between and still contain added preservatives and flavors. So, skip the bottled stuff and instead, brew and ice your own (and add your own sweetener, such as raw honey or stevia).

SWAP SPORTS DRINKS FOR WATER

Though your pediatrician or soccer coach may have advocated them once upon a time, sports drinks aren't much more than colored sugar water with a few electrolytes thrown in. One twenty-ounce (570 ml) bottle contains more than thirty grams of added sugar—which is more added sugar than you should consume in one day.

Water will always be the best thirst quencher. If you're an athlete, consider sipping fresh or unpasteurized coconut water to replenish electrolytes instead of reaching for that sports drink.

Dried Tea

There are many types of tea, and they fall into two categories: pure tea and herbal tea. The main difference is that pure tea contains caffeine, while herbal tea does not. Choosing the best-quality tea is simple with these tips:

1. **Always choose organic to limit chemical exposure.** Tea leaves are heavily sprayed with pesticides, which end up in your cup.

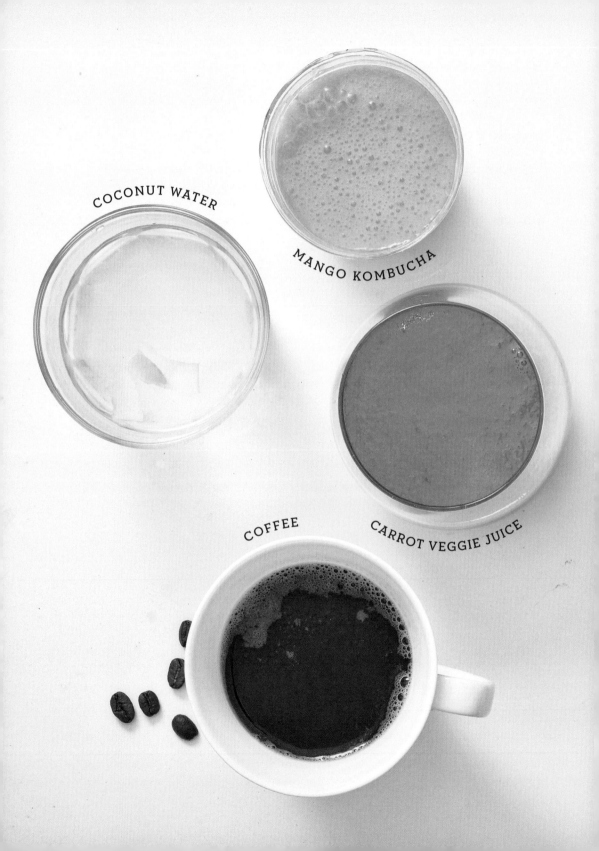

COCONUT WATER

MANGO KOMBUCHA

COFFEE

CARROT VEGGIE JUICE

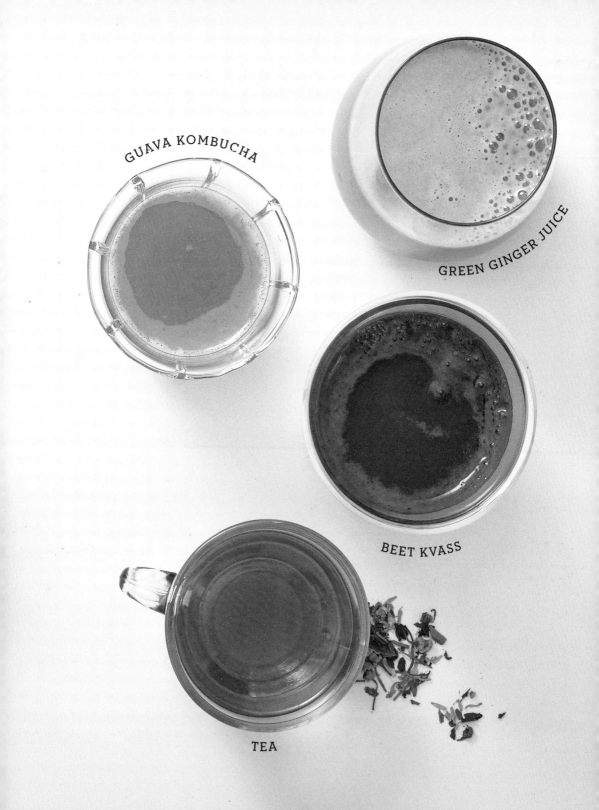

GUAVA KOMBUCHA

GREEN GINGER JUICE

BEET KVASS

TEA

2. **Ideally, choose loose leaf.** Loose tea may contain more antioxidants than tea in teabags because the leaves are less processed. (The actual antioxidant content of tea varies by crop and brand.)

3. **Choose herbal tea to avoid caffeine (optional).** To limit caffeine intake, reach for herbal varieties, such as peppermint or chamomile, instead of pure teas.

Pure Tea

Pure tea—including black, green, white, matcha, Earl Grey, English breakfast, and oolong—all come from the same plant, *Camelia sinesis*, and contain caffeine. What differentiates them is the age of the leaf, how it was grown, and how it was processed. All pure tea contains caffeine. Here are a few of the benefits of drinking each of these teas.

Black Tea

Black tea has high concentrations of the antioxidant compounds known as *theaflavins* and *thearubigins*, which have been linked to lower levels of cholesterol—although green, white, or matcha teas offer more antioxidants and more benefits.

Black tea has a slightly bitter flavor and contains more caffeine than any other tea—about forty milligrams per cup (235 ml). (A cup, or 235 ml, of coffee has 50 to 100 ml.)

Green Tea

Green tea delivers all-around health benefits by the cupful. It's full of antioxidants called *catechins*; a subgroup known as EGCG may ward off everything from cancer to heart disease while helping you burn fat, too. It also contains compounds that help you feel satiated and anti-inflammatory properties that support clear skin.

Green tea has a more delicate flavor than black tea and contains about twenty-five milligrams of caffeine per cup (235 ml).

Oolong Tea

Oolong tea is best known for its support in weight loss. It boosts the metabolism to help you burn fat faster. Studies have shown that drinking oolong tea has led to sustained weight loss and a smaller waist size. In terms of taste, it's similar to black tea, but richer. It contains about thirty milligrams of caffeine per cup (235 ml).

White Tea

White tea is made from the youngest leaves and is the least processed, so it tends to have more antioxidants and a much milder flavor than any other variety, not to mention less caffeine—about fifteen milligrams per cup (235 ml). And, because it has the most antioxidants, it may have more cardiovascular and cancer-fighting benefits than other teas.

Matcha Tea

Bright green matcha powder is the only form of tea in which the whole leaf is consumed (as opposed to being steeped and discarded). Although it contains trace minerals and vitamins, what is most special about matcha is its high EGCG content, about two to three times more than regular green tea, which may offer protection against many kinds of cancer, help prevent cardiovascular disease, slow the aging process, and help the body deal better with stress. EGCG may also reduce harmful cholesterol in the blood, stabilize blood sugar levels, help lower high blood pressure, and enhance the body's resistance to many toxins.

Herbal Tea

Herbal teas are made from flowers, roots, barks, fruits, or seeds and are naturally caffeine free. Examples include peppermint and chamomile tea. There are many interesting blends on the market that do everything from soothe a sore throat to prevent gas to speed up elimination. Of course, you can also find blends that just taste good, too.

There are hundreds of herbal teas. Here are a few of my favorites:

Ginger tea: This tea soothes an upset stomach and supports digestion. Drink it after dinner if you feel bloated or gassy.

Chamomile tea: This is a great option before bed to soothe nerves, release anxiety, and encourage better sleep.

Echinacea tea: Because it supports your immune system, it's wonderful in the winter months when trying to ward off colds and flu.

Peppermint tea: This also supports healthy digestion and soothes an upset stomach. As with ginger tea, drink it after dinner if you feel bloated or gassy.

Coffee

Coffee is one of the most widely consumed morning beverages. Studies suggest that drinking coffee can improve heart health, and the caffeine jolt may sharpen your thinking, boost your metabolism, and improve your physical performance. However, some people are sensitive to caffeine and too much can lead to insomnia, nervousness, and restlessness. If you're a coffee drinker and experience any of these issues, consider cutting back or switching to caffeine-free herbal tea.

But if you love the taste of coffee and don't notice any adverse effects when you drink it, upgrade your brew now! Here's how to choose the healthiest coffee:

1. **Always choose organic.** Coffee is the most heavily pesticide-sprayed food crop in the world!

2. **Ideally, choose shade-grown coffee.** Coffee is a shade-loving shrub and naturally occurring varieties can only be cultivated under a canopy of shade trees. What we now refer to as "shade-grown coffee" was the *only* way coffee was cultivated—until about twenty-five years ago, when new full-sun hybrids were developed that produced substantially higher yields for coffee farmers and allowed the creation of massive agribusiness-style plantations. This comes at the expense of both flavor and the environment. Shade-grown coffee tastes better, is less bitter, and requires less chemical spraying.

CHAPTER 17

MEAT & DAIRY ALTERNATIVES

As a result of plant-based diets becoming ever more popular, dozens of meat, dairy, and animal product alternatives have flooded the market. But, from a health standpoint, some of these are better than others.

Unfortunately, many of these products are highly processed and full of inferior ingredients, such as isolated soy protein, unhealthy oils, and GMO corn. (See "Faux Meat" on page 256.) So, when you're switching to a plant-based diet, remember you don't have to substitute animal products for plant-based products on a one-for-one basis.

For instance, if you usually eat chicken, you don't have to replace it with "fake chicken." Try beans or lentils instead. Or, instead of putting plant-based cheese on a pizza, why not skip the cheese altogether and pile on the veggies and a tapenade? You won't miss a thing.

Still, if these one-for-one swaps help you transition to more plant-based foods, so be it. Just use them sparingly and don't make them dietary staples.

Meat Swaps

Here's what you need to know about plant-based meat and dairy alternatives to make the best choices for a healthy diet.

SWAP MEAT, CHICKEN, & FISH FOR PLANT-BASED ALTERNATIVES

If you want meaty texture without the downsides of processed faux meats, there are great plant-based alternatives made with beans, lentils, quinoa, mushrooms, and tempeh.

Beans & Lentils

Any bean or lentil can be made into patties or processed into a meat-like texture. For example, you can grind cooked kidney beans in a food processor and add steak seasoning for a convincing plant-based "taco meat." Simply sautéed or baked with garlic and spices, beans or lentils also make a hearty alternative to meat.

Quinoa

Quinoa is a complete plant protein, making it an excellent swap for meat. Although it doesn't resemble or taste like meat, it's still filling and satisfying.

Portobello Mushrooms

Portobello mushrooms have a nice, meaty texture and are great for grilling in place of burgers.

Bean or Veggie Burgers

Bean or veggie burgers can be homemade or purchased.

Organic Tempeh

Tempeh is a type of fermented soy that comes in a block and has a neutral flavor, so it can be cut, seasoned, and cooked any way you like. It offers a convincing, meaty texture, too. You'll find it in the refrigerator section. Choose organic to avoid GMOs.

Dairy Swaps

Many nondairy alternatives, particularly milks and cheeses, have a host of ingredients, including those you would not stock in your own kitchen.

But as consumers have begun to demand more whole-food products, there are plenty of options on the market for milks, yogurts, ice creams, and cheeses made simply from nuts, coconut, and vegetables—and they taste just like the real thing. Homemade versions are always best, but when they are not an option, here's how you can choose the healthiest nondairy alternatives:

- **Avoid any milks with carrageenan in the ingredients list.** Carrageenan is a controversial ingredient found to be pro-inflammatory, damaging to the digestive system, and possibly carcinogenic. You'll find it in a variety of nondairy milks—even organic ones—used as a thickener.

- **Choose unsweetened milks to avoid extra sugar.** Choose brands without any sweetener in the ingredients list.

- **Avoid processed soy products.** Soy milk, cheese, and ice cream are heavily processed, which creates a less nutritious and, possibly, harmful product, as discussed in chapter 6. Because it's a controversial ingredient and there are better alternatives, it's best avoided.

- **Avoid casein in nondairy cheese or creamer.** Casein is a dairy protein, so it negates the purpose of a nondairy product!

SWAP BUTTER FOR HEALTHY OILS

Although there are nondairy butters on the market, butter is best replaced with healthy oils, such as olive, avocado, and coconut oils. You could also try coconut butter, which is simply puréed coconut meat; it's rich, creamy, and decadent. Fake butters are typically made from inferior oils and should be avoided.

SWAP CHEESE FOR NONDAIRY CHEESE

Many coconut-, nut-, seed-, and vegetable-based cheeses have entered the market, and they're increasingly getting closer to tasting like the real thing. Health food stores will have the largest selections. The more artisanal brands, which are made simply from fresh nut milks plus enzymes, cultures, and salt, taste the best. The more processed, commercial kinds will have more fillers and additives and tend to taste a little plasticky.

If you try one and don't like it, try another: They vary vastly in taste and texture. Some are made to be sliced and eaten as is, like a European-style cheese, while others are made specifically for melting, so choose the

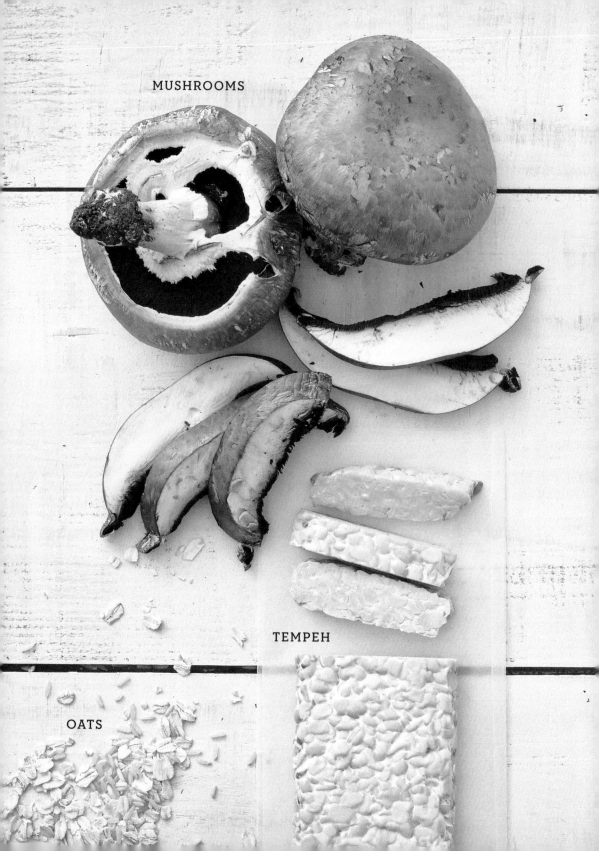

MUSHROOMS

TEMPEH

OATS

KIDNEY BEANS

VEGGIE BURGERS

cheese that fits your style of preparation. But avoid soy cheeses because processed soy is controversial.

SWAP ICE CREAM FOR NONDAIRY ICE CREAM

There are also coconut- and nut-based ice creams on the market, and some are even sweetened with more natural sweeteners. They taste just as good, if not better, than dairy ice creams, so you won't miss a thing. Be warned that some taste better than others, though, so as with other nondairy alternatives, try a few brands to discover which you prefer.

SWAP YOGURT FOR NONDAIRY YOGURT

Like nondairy ice cream, there are many nondairy yogurts on the market, but most are either loaded with sugar or are simply unpalatable. It's better to buy the unflavored varieties and then add your own fruit and nut toppings as you wish to avoid additional refined sugar. You can also find recipes online to make your own from coconut or nuts.

Another good alternative is chia pudding, which has a similar thick, creamy texture. You can find commercial versions, or you can easily make your own: Stir a quarter cup (52 g) chia seeds into one cup (235 ml) coconut milk. Cover and refrigerate overnight.

! Expert Tip

Faux Meat

For many people who embark on a more plant-based diet, their first inclination is to replace chicken with "chick'n." Though most fake meat is not considered "health food," it can be a great way for picky eaters to transition to a more plant-based diet, eventually to be replaced by less processed, more whole-food options, such as quinoa, beans, lentils, split peas, mushrooms, and tempeh.

The following guidelines will help you choose your faux meat wisely:

1. **Avoid soy protein isolate and GMOs:** Most faux meat is made from soy, which is probably GMO if it isn't organic or Non-GMO Project verified. Plus, while traditionally prepared fermented soy is associated with health benefits, the processed soy isolate typically found in faux meat is associated with health concerns. See chapter 6 for more details.

2. **Avoid gluten:** Many meat-based alternatives are made with gluten, which can be inflammatory and is associated with a range of health concerns. For instance, seitan, one particular type of faux meat, is pure wheat gluten.

3. **Watch out for chemicals and fillers:** Check the ingredients list on the back of a faux meat package, and you'll likely see a variety of fillers and chemicals, such as maltodextrin, potassium dichloride, and yeast extract as well as inferior oils, such as canola. These are going to be hard to avoid in faux meat. So, if you're using it as a short-term transition food, choose organic to avoid GMO chemicals and fillers.

CONCLUSION

You've probably heard the phrase "you are what you eat" a million times before—but, by now, I bet you truly understand what it means! Your health is your greatest asset, and now you have the knowledge and tools to take control of it through better food choices.

If the way of eating presented here is starkly different from what you're accustomed to, don't let that overwhelm you. You don't have to completely over-haul your diet overnight—just take one step at a time. It may take you months to convert fully to the real-food way of eating, and that is okay! There's no dogma attached to any of this—and this shouldn't stress you out. When you decide that health is your priority, and that you're worth it, switching to this way of eating becomes easy. You might find it helpful to focus on upgrading one food group at a time, concentrating on it for a week, or even a month, before making changes to another area of your diet.

As you start the switch to real foods, you will feel and look better, and you'll probably want to share it with the world—and you should! The best way to ensure this real-food way of eating becomes a real way of life—not some crash diet—is to share the message you learned here with the people you care about: your family, your friends, and your coworkers.

There's no question that our food is our medicine. So eat as if your life depends on it—because it does!

If you'd like to access bonus content based on this book, go to mariamarlowe.com/real-food-guide for additional chapters covering spices and superfoods, as well as a complete list of specific brand recommendations.

If *The Real Food Grocery Guide* resonated with you and had a positive effect on your eating habits, I'd love to hear from you! Please share your thoughts or success stories with me at: realfood@mariamarlowe.com.

REFERENCES

Chapter 1

Adams, K.M., K.C. Lindell, M. Kohlmeier, and S.H. Zeisel. "Status of Nutrition Education in Medical Schools." *American Journal of Clinical Nutrition* 83, no. 4 (April 2006): 941S–944S. Accessed February 10, 2016. www.ncbi.nlm.nih.gov/pubmed/16600952.

Butler, K. "I Went to the Nutritionists' Annual Confab. It Was Catered by McDonald's." *Mother Jones*. May 12, 2014. Accessed February 10, 2016. www.motherjones.com/environment/2014/05/my-trip-mcdonalds-sponsored-nutritionist-convention.

Hamilton, A. *Squeezed: What You Don't Know About Orange Juice*. New Haven: Yale University Press, 2010.

Harvard T.H. Chan School of Public Health. "Healthy Eating Plate vs. USDA's MyPlate." The Nutrition Source. n.d. Accessed February 10, 2016. www.hsph.harvard.edu/nutritionsource/healthy-eating-plate-vs-usda-myplate/.

Johns, D.J., J. Hartmann-Boyce, S.A. Jebb, and P. Aveyard. "Diet or Exercise Interventions vs. Combined Behavioral Weight Management Programs: A Systematic Review and Meta-Analysis of Direct Comparisons." *Journal of the Academy of Nutrition and Dietetics* 114, no. 10 (October 2014): 1557–1568. doi:10.1016/j.jand.2014.07.005.

Mozaffarian, D., T. Hao, E.B. Rimm, W.C. Willett, and F.B. Hu. "Changes in Diet and Lifestyle and Long-Term Weight Gain in Women and Men." *New England Journal of Medicine* 364, no. 25 (June 2011): 2392–2404. doi:10.1056/NEJMoa1014296.

Rovell, D. *First In Thirst: How Gatorade Turned the Science of Sweat Into a Cultural Phenomenon*. New York: American Management Association, 2005.

Simon, M. "And Now a Word from Our Sponsors: Are America's Nutrition Professionals in the Pocket of Big Food?" *Eat Drink Politics*. 2013. Accessed February 10, 2016. www.eatdrinkpolitics.com/wp-content/uploads/AND_Corporate_Sponsorship_Report.pdf.

Wilks, D.C., S.J. Sharp, U. Ekelund, et al. Gravenor, M., ed. "Objectively Measured Physical Activity and Fat Mass in Children: A Bias-Adjusted Meta-Analysis of Prospective Studies." *PLOS ONE* 6, no. 2 (February 2011): e17205. doi:10.1371/journal.pone.0017205.

Willett, W.C. "Diet and Cancer." *The Oncologist* 5, no. 5 (June 2000): 393–404. doi:10.1634/theoncologist.5-5-393.

Chapter 2

Adebamowo, C.A., D. Spiegelman, F.W. Danby, A.L. Frazier, W.C. Willett, and M.D. Holmes. "High School Dietary Dairy Intake and Teenage Acne." *Journal of the American Academy of Dermatology* 52, no. 2 (February 2005): 207–214. doi:10.1016/j.jaad.2004.08.007.

Agrawal, R., and F. Gomez-Pinilla. "'Metabolic Syndrome' in the Brain: Deficiency in Omega-3 Fatty Acid Exacerbates Dysfunctions in Insulin Receptor Signalling and Cognition." *Journal of Physiology* 590, no. 10 (May 2012): 2485–2499. doi:10.1113/jphysiol.2012.230078.

Anand, P., A.B. Kunnumakkara, C. Sundaram, et al. "Cancer is a Preventable Disease that Requires Major Lifestyle Changes." *Pharmaceutical Research* 25, no. 9 (September 2008): 2097–2116. doi:10.1007/s11095-008-9661-9.

Burris, J., W. Rietkerk, and K. Woolf. "Acne: The Role of Medical Nutrition Therapy." *Journal of the Academy of Nutrition and Dietetics* 113, no. 3 (March 2013): 416–430. doi:10.1016/j.jand.2012.11.016.

Chew, E.Y., T.E. Clemons, E. Agrón, L.J. Launer, F. Grodstein, and P.S. Bernstein. "Effect of Omega-3 Fatty Acids, Lutein/Zeaxanthin, or Other Nutrient Supplementation on Cognitive Function." *Journal of the American Medical Association* 314, no. 8 (August 2015): 791–801. doi:10.1001/jama.2015.9677.

Kerti, L., A.V. Witte, A. Winkler, U. Grittner, D. Rujescu, and A. Flöel. "Higher Glucose Levels Associated with Lower Memory and Reduced Hippocampal

Microstructure." *Neurology* 81, no. 20 (November 2013): 1746–1752. doi:10.1212/01.wnl.0000435561.00234.ee.

Magnusson, K.R., L. Hauck, B.M. Jeffrey, et al. "Relationships Between Diet-Related Changes in the Gut Microbiome and Cognitive Flexibility." *Neuroscience* 300 (August 2015): 128–140. Accessed February 10, 2016. http://dx.doi.org/10.1016/j.neuroscience.2015.05.016.

Maki, J. "Berries Keep Your Brain Sharp." *Harvard Gazette*. April 26, 2012. Accessed February 10, 2016. http://news.harvard.edu/gazette/story/2012/04/berries-keep-your-brain-sharp/.

Ornish, D., L.W. Scherwitz, J.H. Billings, et al. "Intensive Lifestyle Changes for Reversal of Coronary Heart Disease." *Journal of the American Medical Association* 280, no. 23 (December 1998): 2001–2007. doi:10.1001/jama.280.23.2001.

Smith, R.N., N.J. Mann, A. Braue, H. Mäkeläinen, and G.A. Varigos. "A Low Glycemic-Load Diet Improves Symptoms in Acne Vulgaris Patients: A Randomized Controlled Trial." *American Journal of Clinical Nutrition* 86, no. 1 (July 2007): 107–115. Accessed February 10, 2016. http://ajcn.nutrition.org/content/86/1/107.full#aff-1.

Wolpert, S. "Scientists Learn How What You Eat Affects Your Brain—and Those of Your Kids." *UCLA Newsroom*. July 9, 2008. Accessed February 10, 2016. http://newsroom.ucla.edu/releases/scientists-learn-how-food-affects-52668.

Wu, S., S. Powers, W. Zhu, and Y.A. Hannun. "Substantial Contribution of Extrinsic Risk Factors to Cancer Development." *Nature* 529, no. 7584 (January 2016): 43–47. doi:10.1038/nature16166.

Chapter 4

Barański, M., D. Średnicka-Tober, N. Volakakis, et al. "Higher Antioxidant and Lower Cadmium Concentrations and Lower Incidence of Pesticide Residues in Organically Grown Crops: A Systematic Literature Review and Meta-Analyses." *British Journal of Nutrition* 112, no. 5 (September 2014): 794–811. doi:10.1017/S0007114514001366.

Cosgrove, M.C., O.H. Franco, S.P. Granger, P.G. Murray, and A.E. Mayes. "Dietary Nutrient Intakes and Skin-Aging Appearance Among Middle-Aged American Women." *American Journal of Clinical Nutrition* 86, no. 4 (October 2007): 1225–1231. Accessed February 10, 2016. http://ajcn.nutrition.org/content/86/4/1225.long.

Fenwick, G.R., and R.K. Heaney. "Glucosinolates and Their Breakdown Products in Cruciferous Crops, Foods, and Feedingstuffs." *Critical Reviews in Food Science and Nutrition* 18, no. 2 (January 1983): 123–201. doi:10.1016/0308-8146(83)90074-2.

Fleischauer, A.T., and L. Arab. "Garlic and Cancer: A Critical Review of the Epidemiologic Literature." *Journal of Nutrition* 131, no. 3s (March 2001): 1032S–1040S. Accessed February 10, 2016. www.ncbi.nlm.nih.gov/pubmed/11238811.

Fujioka, K., F. Greenway, J. Sheard, and Y. Ying. "The Effects of Grapefruit on Weight and Insulin Resistance: Relationship to the Metabolic Syndrome." *Journal of Medicinal Food* 9, no. 1 (March 2006): 49–54. doi:10.1089/jmf.2006.9.49.

Giovannucci, E. "Tomatoes, tomato-based products, lycopene, and cancer: review of the epidemiologic literature," *Journal of the National Cancer Institute*. February 17, 1999;91(4):317–331.

Hecht, S.S. "Chemoprevention by Isothiocyanates." *Journal of Cellular Biochemistry* 59, Sup S22 (1995): 195–209. Accessed February 10, 2016. doi:10.1002/jcb.240590825.

Higdon, J.V., B. Delage, D.E. Williams, and R.H. Dashwood. "Cruciferous Vegetables and Human Cancer Risk: Epidemiologic Evidence and Mechanistic Basis." *Pharmacological Research* 55, no. 3 (March 2007): 224–236. doi:10.1016/j.phrs.2007.01.009.

Kang, J.H., A. Ascherio, and F. Grodstein. "Fruit and Vegetable Consumption and Cognitive Decline in Aging Women." *Annals of Neurology* 57, no. 5 (May 2005): 713–720. doi:10.1002/ana.20476.

Lampe, J.W., and S. Peterson. "Brassica, Biotransformation, and Cancer Risk: Genetic Polymorphisms Alter the Preventive Effects of Cruciferous Vegetables." *Journal of Nutrition* 132, no. 10 (October 2002): 2991–2994. Accessed February 10, 2016. http://jn.nutrition.org/content/132/10/2991.full.

Lin, B.H., and R.M. Morrison. "Higher Fruit Consumption Linked with Lower Body Mass Index." *Food Review* 25 (2002): 28–32. Accessed February 10, 2016. www.andeal.org/worksheet.cfm?worksheet_id=115541.

Muggeridge, D.J., C.C. Howe, O. Spendiff, C. Pedlar, P.E. James, and C. Easton. "A Single Dose of Beetroot Juice Enhances Cycling Performance in Simulated Altitude." *Medicine and Science in Sports and*

Exercise 46, no. 1 (January 2014): 143–150. doi:10.1249/MSS.0b013e3182a1dc51.

Nakamura, Y., and N. Miyoshi. "Cell Death Induction by Isothiocyanates and their Underlying Molecular Mechanisms." *BioFactors* 26, no. 2 (2006): 123–134. Accessed February 10, 2016. www.ncbi.nlm.nih.gov/pubmed/16823098.

National Cancer Institute. "Usual Dietary Intakes: Food Intakes, U.S. Population, 2007–10." *Epidemiology and Genomics Research Program.* Accessed February 10, 2016. http://epi.grants.cancer.gov/diet/usualintakes/pop/2007-10/.

Okeniyi, J.A., T.A. Ogunlesi, O.A. Oyelami, and L.A. Adeyemi. "Effectiveness of Dried Carica Papaya Seeds Against Human Intestinal Parasitosis: A Pilot Study." *Journal of Medicinal Food* 10, no. 1 (May 2007): 194–196. doi:10.1089/jmf.2005.065.

Oude Griep, L.M., W.M. Verschuren, D. Kromhout, M.C. Océ, and J.M. Geleijnse. "Colours of Fruit and Vegetables and Ten-Year Incidence of CHD. *British Journal of Nutrition* 106, no. 10 (November 2011): 1562–1569. doi:10.1017/S0007114511001942.

Oyebode, O., V. Gordon-Dseagu, A. Walker, and J.S. Mindell. "Fruit and Vegetable Consumption and All-Cause, Cancer, and CVD Mortality: Analysis of Health Survey for England Data." *BMJ Journal of Epidemiology and Community Health* 68, no. 9 (September 2014): 856–862. doi:10.1136/jech-2013-203500.

Palomo, I., E. Fuentes, T. Padró, and L. Badimon. "Platelets and atherogenesis: Platelet anti-aggregation activity and endothelial protection from tomatoes (*Solanum lycopersicum* L.)," *Experimental and Therapeutic Medicine*, April 2012;3(4): 577–584.

Perego, P., L. Gatti, N. Carenini, L. Dal Bo, and F. Zunino. "Apoptosis Induced by Extracellular Glutathione Is Mediated by H2O2 Production and DNA Damage." *International Journal of Cancer* 87, no. 3 (July 2000): 343–348. doi:10.1002/1097-0215(20000801)87:3<343::AID-IJC6>3.0.CO;2-8.

Presley, T.D., A.R. Morgan, E. Bechtold, et al. "Acute Effect of a High Nitrate Diet on Brain Perfusion in Older Adults." *Nitric Oxide: Biology and Chemistry* 24, no. 1 (January 2011): 34–42. doi:10.1016/j.niox.2010.10.002.

Purba, M.B., A. Kouris-Blazos, N. Wattanapenpaiboon, et al. "Skin Wrinkling: Can Food Make a Difference?" *Journal of the American College of Nutrition* 20, no. 1

(February 2001): 71–80. Accessed February 10, 2016. www.ncbi.nlm.nih.gov/pubmed/11293471.

Schroder, K.E. "Effects of Fruit Consumption on Body Mass Index and Weight Loss in a Sample of Overweight and Obese Dieters Enrolled in a Weight-Loss Intervention Trial." *Nutrition* 26, nos. 7–8 (July–August 2010): 727–734. doi:10.1016/j.nut.2009.08.009.

Song, K., and J.A. Milner. "The Influence of Heating on the Anticancer Properties of Garlic." *Journal of Nutrition* 131, no. 3s (March 2001): 1054S–1057S. Accessed February 10, 2016. www.ncbi.nlm.nih.gov/pubmed/11238815.

Takezaki, T., C-M. Gao, J-H. Ding, T-K. Liu, M-S. Li, and K. Tajima. "Comparative Study of Lifestyles of Residents in High- and Low-Risk Areas for Gastric Cancer in Jiangsu Province, China; with Special Reference to Allium Vegetables." *Journal of Epidemiology.* 9, no. 5 (November 1999): 297–305. doi:10.2188/jea.9.297.

Truong, T., D. Baron-Dubourdieu, Y. Rougier, and P. Guénel. "Role of Dietary Iodine and Cruciferous Vegetables in Thyroid Cancer: A Countrywide Case-Control Study in New Caledonia." *Cancer Causes and Control* 21, no. 8 (August 2010): 1183–1192. doi:10.1007/s10552-010-9545-2.

University of Maine. "Best Ways to Wash Fruits and Vegetables." Accessed February 10, 2016. http://umaine.edu/publications/4336e/.

University of Maryland Medical Center. "Manganese." *Complementary and Alternative Medicine Guide.* Supplement. Accessed March 28, 2016. http://umm.edu/health/medical/altmed/supplement/manganese.

U.S. 2010 Dietary Guidelines. Accessed February 10, 2016. http://health.gov/dietaryguidelines/2010/.

U.S. Dietary Guidelines 2015–2020, 8th ed. Accessed February 10, 2016. http://health.gov/dietaryguidelines/2015/guidelines/.

Verhoeven, D.T.H., R.A. Goldbohm, G. van Poppel, H. Verhagen, and P.A. van den Brandt. "Epidemiological Studies on Brassica Vegetables and Cancer Risk." *Cancer Epidemiology, Biomarkers, & Prevention* 5, no. 9 (October 1996): 733–748. Accessed February 10, 2016. www.researchgate.net/publication/14329966_Epidemiological_studies_on_brassica_vegetables_and_cancer_risk_Cancer_Epidemiol_Biomarkers_Prev_5733-748.

What's On My Food? "Pesticides on Apples." Accessed February 10, 2016. www.whatsonmyfood.org/food.jsp?food=ap.

Zhang, Y., S. Yao, and J. Li. "Vegetable-Derived Isothiocyanates: Anti-proliferative Activity and Mechanism in Action." *Proceedings of the Nutrition Society* 65, no. 1 (February 2006): 68–75. Accessed February 10, 2016. www.ncbi.nlm.nih.gov/pubmed/16441946.

Chapter 5

Specter, M. "Against the Grain." *New Yorker*. November 3, 2014. Accessed February 10, 2016. www.newyorker.com/magazine/2014/11/03/grain.

Yang, L., J.D. Browning, and J.M. Awika. "Sorghum 3-Deoxyanthocyanins Possess Strong Phase II Enzyme Inducer Activity and Cancer Cell Growth Inhibition Properties." *Journal of Agricultural and Food Chemistry* 57, no. 5 (March 2009): 1797–1804. Accessed February 10, 2016. www.ncbi.nlm.nih.gov/pubmed/19256554.

Chapter 6

Aune, D., E. DeStefani, A. Ronco, et al. "Legume Intake and the Risk of Cancer: A Multisite Case-Control Study in Uruguay." *Cancer Causes and Control* 20, no. 9 (November 2009): 1605–1615. doi:10.1007/s10552-009-9406-z.

Bazzano, L.A., J. He, L.G. Ogden, et al. "Legume Consumption and Risk of Coronary Heart Disease in U.S. Men and Women." *Archives of Internal Medicine* 161, no. 21 (December 2001): 2573–2578. doi:10.1001/archinte.161.21.2573.

Dewell, A., G. Weidner, M.D. Sumner, et al. "Relationship of Dietary Protein and Soy Isoflavones to Serum IGF-1 and IGF Binding Proteins in the Prostate Cancer Lifestyle Trial." *Nutrition and Cancer* 58, no. 1 (2007): 35–42. Accessed February 10, 2016. doi:10.1080/01635580701308034.

Ha, V., J.L. Sievenpiper, R.J. de Souza, et al. "Effect of Dietary Pulse Intake on Established Therapeutic Lipid Targets for Cardiovascular Risk Reduction: A Systematic Review and Meta-Analysis of Randomized Controlled Trials." *Canadian Medical Association Journal* (April 2014). Accessed February 10, 2016. doi:10.1503/cmaj.131727.

Harvard T.H. Chan School of Public Health. "Protein." *The Nutrition Source*. Accessed February 10, 2016. www.hsph.harvard.edu/nutritionsource/what-should-you-eat/protein/.

Heaney, R.P., D.A. McCarron, B. Dawson-Hughes, et al. "Dietary Changes Favorably Affect Bone Remodeling in Older Adults." *Journal of the Academy of Nutrition and Dietetics* 99, no. 10 (October 1999): 1228–1233. Accessed February 10, 2016. doi:http://dx.doi.org/10.1016/S0002-8223(99)00302-8.

Jenkins, D.J, C.W. Kendall, L.S. Augustin, et al. "Effect of Legumes as Part of a Low Glycemic Index Diet on Glycemic Control and Cardiovascular Risk Factors in Type 2 Diabetes Mellitus: A Randomized Controlled Trial." *Journal of the American Medical Association Archives of Internal Medicine* 172, no. 21 (November 2012): 1653–1660. doi:10.1001/2013.jamainternmed.70.

Jenkins, D.J., A. Mirrahimi, K. Srichaikul, et al. "Soy Protein Reduces Serum Cholesterol by Both Intrinsic and Food Displacement Mechanisms." *Journal of Nutrition* 140, no. 12 (December 2010): 2302S–2311S. doi:10.3945/jn.110.124958.

McCullough, M. "The Bottom Line on Soy and Breast Cancer Risk." *Expert Voices Blog*. August 2, 2012. Accessed February 10, 2016. http://blogs.cancer.org/expertvoices/2012/08/02/the-bottom-line-on-soy-and-breast-cancer-risk/?

Messina, M. "Soybean Isoflavone Exposure Does Not Have Feminizing Effects on Men: A Critical Examination of the Clinical Evidence." *Fertility and Sterility* 93, no. 7 (May 2010): 2095–2104. doi:10.1016/j.fertnstert.2010.03.002.

Messina, M., and G. Redmond. "Effects of Soy Protein and Soybean Isoflavones on Thyroid Function in Healthy Adults and Hypothyroid Patients: A Review of the Relevant Literature." *Thyroid* 16, no. 3 (March 2006): 249–258. Accessed February 10, 2016. doi:10.1089/thy.2006.16.249.

Physicians Committee for Responsible Medicine. "Soy and Your Health." Accessed February 10, 2016. www.pcrm.org/health/health-topics/soy-and-your-health.

Shu, X.O., Y. Zheng, H. Cai, Z. Chen, W. Zheng, and W. Lu. "Soy Food Intake and Breast Cancer Survival." *Journal of the American Medical Association* 302, no. 22 (December 2009): 2437–2443. doi:10.1001/jama.2009.1783.

Chapter 7

Abbas, H.K. *Aflatoxin and Food Safety*. Boca Raton, Florida: CRC Taylor & Francis, 2005.

Bes-Rastrollo, M., N.M. Wedick, M.A. Martinez-Gonzalez, T.Y. Li, L. Sampson, and F.B. Hu. "Prospective Study of Nut Consumption, Long-Term Weight Change, and Obesity Risk in Women." *American Journal of Clinical Nutrition* 89, no. 6 (June 2009): 1913–1919. doi:10.3945/ajcn.2008.27276.

Josse, A.R., C.W. Kendall, L.S. Augustin, P.R. Ellis, and D.J. Jenkins. "Almonds and Postprandial Glycemia—A Dose-Response Study." *Metabolism* 56, no. 3 (March 2007): 400–404. doi:10.1016/j.metabol.2006.10.024.

Jubert, C., J. Mata, G. Bench, et al. "Effects of Chlorophyll and Chlorophyllin on Low-Dose Aflatoxin B1 Pharmacokinetics in Human Volunteers." *Cancer Prevention Research* 2, no. 12 (December 2009): 1015–1022. doi:10.1158/1940-6207.CAPR-09-0099.

López-González, A.A., F. Grases, P. Roca, B. Mari, M.T. Vicente-Herrero, and A. Costa-Bauzá. "Phytate (Myo-Inositol Hexaphosphate) and Risk Factors for Osteoporosis." *Journal of Medicinal Food* 11, no. 4 (December 2008): 747–752. doi:10.1089/jmf.2008.0087.

Mattes, R.D., and M.L. Dreher. "Nuts and Healthy Body Weight Maintenance Mechanisms." *Asia Pacific Journal of Clinical Nutrition* 19, no. 1 (2010): 137–41. Accessed February 10, 2010. www.ncbi.nlm.nih.gov/pubmed/20199999.

Moss, M. "Are Nuts a Weight-Loss Aid?" *New York Times*. December 17, 2013. Accessed February 10, 2016. www.nytimes.com/2013/12/18/dining/are-nuts-a-weight-loss-aid.html.

Puangsombat, K., and J.S. Smith. "Inhibition of Heterocyclic Amine Formation in Beef Patties by Ethanolic Extracts of Rosemary." *Journal of Food Science* 75, no. 2 (March 2010): T40–T47. doi:10.1111/j.1750-3841.2009.01491.x.

Unnevehr, L.J., and D. Grace. *Aflatoxins: Finding Solutions for Improved Food Safety*. Washington, D.C.: International Food Policy Research Institute, 2013.

Wien, M.A., J.M. Sabaté, D.N. Iklé, and F.R. Kandeel. "Almonds vs. Complex Carbohydrates in a Weight Reduction Program." *International Journal of Obesity and Related Metabolic Disorders* 27, no. 11 (November 2003): 1365–1372. Accessed February 10, 2016. www.ncbi.nlm.nih.gov/pubmed/14574348.

Williams, J.H., T.D. Phillips, P.E. Jolly, J.K. Stiles, C.M. Jolly, and D. Aggarwal. "Human Aflatoxicosis in Developing Countries: A Review of Toxicology, Exposure, Potential Health Consequences, and Interventions." *American Journal of Clinical Nutrition* 80, no. 5 (November 2004): 1106–1122. Accessed February 10, 2016. http://ajcn.nutrition.org/content/80/5/1106.long.

Chapter 8

Centers for Disease Control and Prevention. "Antibiotic Resistance and Food Safety: Frequently Asked Questions." 2015. Accessed February 10, 2016. www.cdc.gov/narms/faq.html.

Govender, S. "These American Meat Products are Banned Abroad." *The Huffington Post* "The BLOG." 2014. Accessed February 10, 2016. www.huffingtonpost.com/the-daily meal/these-american-meat-produ_b_5153275.html.

Pan, A., Q. Sun, A.M. Bernstein, et al. "Red Meat Consumption and Mortality: Results from Two Prospective Cohort Studies." *Archives of Internal Medicine* 172, no. 7 (April 2012): 555–563. doi:10.1001/archinternmed.2011.2287.

U.S. Food and Drug Administration. *2010 Retail Meat Report*. Rockville, MD: U.S. Food and Drug Administration, 2010.

Chapter 9

Barrionuevo, A. "Salmon Virus Indicts Chile's Fishing Methods." *New York Times*. March 27, 2008. Accessed February 20, 2016. www.nytimes.com/2008/03/27/world/americas/27salmon.html.

Baxter, M.R. "The Welfare Problems of Laying Hens in Battery Cages." *The Veterinary Record* 134, no. 24 (June 1994): 614–9. www.ncbi.nlm.nih.gov/pubmed/7941260.

Done, H.Y., and R.U. Halden. "Reconnaissance of 47 Antibiotics and Associated Microbial Risks in Seafood Sold in the United States." *Journal of Hazardous Materials* 282 (January 2015): 10–17. doi:10.1016/j.jhazmat.2014.08.075.

Environmental Working Group. "PCBs in Farmed Salmon." July 31, 2003. Accessed February 10, 2016. www.ewg.org/research/pcbs-farmed-salmon.

Mittelmark, J., and A. Kapuscinski. "Induced Reproduction in Fish." *Minnesota Sea Grant*. 2013. Accessed February 10, 2016. www.seagrant.umn.edu/aquaculture/induced_fish_reproduction.

Chapter 10

Serbe, L., and E. Main. "The Truth About Your Eggs." *ABC News*. July 28, 2012. Accessed February 10, 2016. http://abcnews.go.com/health/truth-eggs/story?id=16871055.

Woodward, M.J., and S.E. Kirwan. "Detection of Salmonella Enteritidis in Eggs by the Polymerase Chain Reaction." *The Veterinary Record* 138, no. 17 (April 1996): 411–13. www.ncbi.nlm.nih.gov/pubmed/8733179.

Chapter 11

Adebamowo, C.A., D. Spiegelman, F.W. Danby, A.L. Frazier, W.C. Willett, and M.D. Holmes. "High School Dietary Dairy Intake and Teenage Acne." *Journal of the American Academy of Dermatology* 52, no. 2 (February 2005): 207–214. Accessed February 10, 2016. doi:10.1016/j.jaad.2004.08.007.

Chan, J.M., M.J, Stampfer, J. Ma, U. Ajani, J.M. Gaziano, and E. Giovannucci. "Dairy Products, Calcium, and Prostate Cancer Risk in the Physicians' Health Study." Presentation. *American Association for Cancer Research* (April 2000).

Cuatrecasas, P., D.H. Lockwood, and J.R. Caldwell. "Lactase Deficiency in the Adult." *The Lancet* 285, no. 7375 (January 1965): 14–18. doi:10.1016/S0140-6736(65)90922-0.

Genkinger, J.M., D.J. Hunter, D. Spiegelman, et al. "Dairy Products and Ovarian Cancer: A Pooled Analysis of 12 Cohort Studies." *Cancer Epidemiology, Biomarkers, and Prevention* 15, no. 2 (February 2006): 364–72. doi:10.1158/1055-9965.EPI-05-0484.

Giovannucci, E., E.B. Rimm, A. Ascherio, et al. "Calcium and Fructose Intake in Relation to Risk of Prostate Cancer." *Cancer Research* 58, no. 3 (February 1998): 442–447. Accessed February 10, 2016. http://cancerres.aacrjournals.org/content/58/3/442.long.

Hebeisen, D.F., F. Hoeflin, H.P. Reusch, E. Junker, and B. Lauterburg. "Increased Concentrations of Omega-3 Fatty Acids in Milk and Platelet Rich Plasma of Grass-Fed Cows." *International Journal for Vitamin and Nutrition Research* 63, no. 6 (February 1993): 229–233. Accessed February 10, 2016. http://bit.ly/1UdVLi8.

Huang, S.S., and T.M. Bayless. "Milk and Lactose Intolerance in Healthy Orientals." *Science* 160, no. 3823 (May 1968): 83–84. doi:10.1126/science.160.3823.83-a.

Kratz, M., T. Baars, and S. Guyenet. "The Relationship Between High-Fat Dairy Consumption and Obesity, Cardiovascular, and Metabolic Disease." *European Journal of Nutrition* 52, no. 1 (February 2013): 1–24. doi:10.1007/s00394-012-0418-1.

Manson, J.E., J. Hsia, K.C. Johnson, et. al. "Estrogen plus Progestin and the Risk of Coronary Heart Disease." *New England Journal of Medicine* 349, no.6 (August 2003): 523–534. Accessed February 10, 2016. doi:10.1056/NEJMoa030808.

Mishkin, S. "Dairy Sensitivity, Lactose Malabsorption, and Elimination Diets in Inflammatory Bowel Disease." *American Journal of Clinical Nutrition* 65, no. 2 (February 1997): 564–567. Accessed February 10, 2016. www.ncbi.nlm.nih.gov/pubmed/9022546.

Moran, B. "Is Butter Really Back?" *Harvard T.H. Chan School of Public Health.* Accessed February 10, 2016. www.hsph.harvard.edu/magazine-features/is-butter-really back/.

Robbins, J. "The Truth About Calcium and Osteoporosis." *Food Matters*. November 2009. Accessed February 10, 2016. http://foodmatters.tv/articles-1/the-truth-about-calcium-and-osteoporosis.

Scharf, R.J., R.T. Demmer, and M.D. DeBoer. "Longitudinal Evaluation of Milk Type Consumed and Weight Status in Preschoolers." *Archives of Disease in Childhood* 98, no. 5 (2013): 335–340. doi:10.1136/archdischild-2012-302941.

Scrimshaw, N.S., and E.B. Murray. "The Acceptability of Milk and Milk Products in Populations with a High Prevalence of Lactose Intolerance." *American Journal of Clinical Nutrition* 48, no. 4 Supplement (October 1988): 1079–1159. Accessed February 10, 2016. www.ncbi.nlm.nih.gov/pubmed/3140651.

Woteki, C.E., E. Weser, and E.A. Young. "Lactose Malabsorption in Mexican-American Children." *American Journal of Clinical Nutrition* 29, no. 1 (January 1976): 19–24. Accessed February 10, 2016. www.ncbi.nlm.nih.gov/pubmed/946157.

Chapter 12

Arnold, L.E., N. Lofthouse, and E. Hurt. "Artificial Food Colors and Attention-Deficit/Hyperactivity Symptoms: Conclusions to Dye For." *Neurotherapeutics* 9, no. 3 (July 2012): 599–609. doi:10.1007/s13311-012-0133-x.

Bae, S., and Y-C. Hong. "Exposure to Bisphenol A from Drinking Canned Beverages Increases Blood Pressure: Randomized Crossover Trial." *Hypertension* 65, no. 2 (February 2015): 313–319. doi:10.1161/HYPERTENSIONAHA.114.04261.

Ballmaier, D., and B. Epe. "Oxidative DNA Damage Induced by Potassium Bromate Under Cell-Free Conditions and in Mammalian Cells." *Carcinogenesis* 16, no. 2 (February 1995): 335–342. doi:10.1093/carcin/16.2.335.

Barnes, J.N., and M.J. Joyner. "Sugar Highs and Lows: The Impact of Diet on Cognitive Function." *Journal of Physiology* 590, no. 12 (June 2012): 2831. doi:10.1113/jphysiol.2012.234328.

Basu, S., P. Yoffe, N. Hills, and R.H. Lustig. "The Relationship of Sugar to Population-Level Diabetes Prevalence: An Econometric Analysis of Repeated Cross-Sectional Data." *PLOS ONE* 8, no. 2 (February 2013). doi:10.1371/journal.pone.0057873.

Benbrook, C.M. "Impacts of Genetically Engineered Crops on Pesticide Use in the U.S.—The First Sixteen Years." *Environmental Sciences Europe* 24, no. 24 (2012). doi:10.1186/2190-4715-24-24.

Burdock, G.A. *Fenaroli's Handbook of Flavor Ingredients*. Boca Raton, Florida: CRC Press, 2005.

Center for Science in the Public Interest. "Regulatory Comment Submitted to the FDA April 2015: Re: Substances Generally Recognized as Safe (GRAS)." Pages 7–8. Accessed March 15, 2016. http://cspinet.org/sites/default/files/attachment/GRAS%20Comment%20FINAL_O.pdf.

Congleton, J. "Propyl Paraben: Are You Eating An Endocrine Disruptor?" *Environmental Working Group*. April 2015. Accessed February 10, 2016. www.ewg.org/research/propyl-paraben.

DiNicolantonio, J.J., and S.C. Lucan. "The Wrong White Crystals: Not Salt but Sugar as Aetiological in Hypertension and Cardiometabolic Disease." *Open Heart* 1, no. 1 (2014). doi:10.1136/openhrt-2014-000167.

Ebbeling, C.B., J.F. Swain, H.A. Feldman, et al. "Effects of Dietary Composition on Energy Expenditure During Weight-Loss Maintenance." *Journal of the American Medical Association* 307, no. 24 (June 2012): 2627–2634. doi:10.1001/jama.2012.6607.

Fernandez-Cornejo, J., and M.F. Caswell. *Genetically Engineered Crops in the United States*. Washington, D.C.: U.S. Dept. of Agriculture, Economic Research Service, 2014.

Festi, D., A. Colecchia, M. Orsini, et al. "Gallbladder Motility and Gallstone Formation in Obese Patients Following Very Low Calorie Diets. Use It (Fat) to Lose It (Well)." *International Journal of Obesity and Related Metabolic Disorders* 22, no. 6 (June 1998): 592–600. Accessed February 10, 2016. www.ncbi.nlm.nih.gov/pubmed/9665682.

Gies, E. "Substitutes for Bisphenol A Could Be More Harmful." *New York Times*. April 18, 2011. Accessed February 10, 2016. www.nytimes.com/2011/04/18/business/global/18iht-rbog-plastic-18.html?_r=0.

Harvard Health Publications, Harvard Medical School. "What You Eat Can Fuel or Cool Inflammation: Body's Response System Key Driver of Heart Disease, Diabetes, and other Chronic Conditions." *The Family Health Guide*. February 2007 Update. Accessed February 10, 2016. www.health.harvard.edu/family_health_guide/what-you-eat-can-fuel-or-cool-inflammation-a-key-driver-of-heart-disease-diabetes-and-other-chronic-conditions.

He, K., S. Du, P. Xun, et al. "Consumption of Monosodium Glutamate in Relation to Incidence of Overweight in Chinese Adults: China Health and Nutrition Survey (CHNS)." *American Journal of Clinical Nutrition* 93, no. 6 (April 2011): 1328–1336. doi:10.3945/ajcn.110.008870.

Humphries, P., E. Pretorius, and H. Naudé. "Direct and Indirect Cellular Effects of Aspartame on the Brain." *European Journal of Clinical Nutrition* 62, no. 4 (April 2008): 451–462. Accessed February 10, 2016. doi:10.1038/sj.ejcn.1602866.

Kobylewski, S., and M.F. Jacobson. *Food Dyes: A Rainbow of Risks*. Washington, D.C.: Center for Science in the Public Interest. June 2010. Accessed February 10, 2016. http://cspinet.org/new/pdf/food-dyes-rainbow-risks.pdf.

Kurokawa, Y., A. Maekawa, M. Takahashi, and Y. Hayashi. "Toxicity and Carcinogenicity of Potassium Bromate—A New Renal Carcinogen." *Environmental Health Perspectives* 87 (July 1990): 309–335. Accessed February 10, 2016. www.ncbi.nlm.nih.gov/pmc/articles/PMC1567851/.

Lustig, R.H. "Sugar: The Bitter Truth." *UCSF Mini Medical School*. Accessed February 2016. www.youtube.com/watch?v=dBnniua6-oM

McCann, D., A. Barrett, A. Cooper, et al. "Food Additives and Hyperactive Behaviour in 3-Year-Old and 8/9-Year-Old Children in the Community: A Randomised, Double-Blinded, Placebo-Controlled Trial." *The Lancet* 370, no. 9598 (November 2007): 1560–1567. doi:10.1016/S0140-6736(07)61306-3.

Neltner, T.G., N.R. Kulkarni, H.M. Alger, et al. "Navigating the U.S. Food Additive Regulatory Program." *Comprehensive Reviews in Food Science and Food Safety* 10, no. 6 (November 2011): 342–368. doi:10.1111/j.1541-4337.2011.00166.x.

Nöthlings, U., L.R. Wilkens, S.P. Murphy, J.H. Hankin, B.E. Henderson, and L.N. Kolonel. "Meat and Fat Intake as Risk Factors for Pancreatic Cancer: The Multiethnic Cohort Study." *Journal of the National Cancer Institute* 97, no. 19 (October 2005): 1458–1465. doi:10.1093/jnci/dji292.

O'Keefe, S., S. Gaskins-Wright, V. Wiley, and I-C. Chen. "Levels of Trans Geometrical Isomers of Essential Fatty Acids in Some Unhydrogenated U.S. Vegetable Oils." *Journal of Food Lipids* 1, no. 3 (September 1994): 165–176. doi:10.1111/j.1745-4522.1994.tb00244.x.

Oishi, S. "Effects of Propyl Paraben on the Male Reproductive System." *Food and Chemical Toxicology* 40, no. 12 (December 2002): 1807–1813. doi: 10.1016/S0278-6915(02)00204-1.

Pan, S., C. Yuan, A. Tagmount, et al. "Parabens and Human Epidermal Growth Factor Receptor Ligands Cross-Talk in Breast Cancer Cells." *Environmental Health Perspectives* 124, no. 5 (May 2016): 563–569. doi:10.1289/ehp.1409200.

Robinson, C., M. Antoniou, and J. Fagan. *GMO Myths and Truths: An Evidence-Based Examination of the Claims Made for the Safety and Efficacy of Genetically Modified Crops and Foods.* 2nd ed. London, Great Britain: Earth Open Source, 2014.

Skerrett, P.J. "Panel Suggests that Dietary Guidelines Stop Warning About Cholesterol in Food." *Harvard Health Publications.* February 12, 2015. Accessed February 10, 2016. http://bit.ly/1kt6nlv.

Smith, J., and S. Seneff. "Jeffrey Smith Interviews Dr. Stephanie Seneff About Glyphosate." *Vimeo.* Accessed February 10, 2016. https://vimeo.com/65914121.

Smith, K.W., I. Souter, I. Dimitriadis, et al. "Urinary Paraben Concentrations and Ovarian Aging Among Women from a Fertility Center." *Environmental Health Perspectives* 121, nos. 11–12 (November–December 2013): 1299–1305. doi:10.1289/ehp.1205350.

Te Morenga, S. Mallard, and J. Mann. "Dietary Sugars and Body Weight: Systematic Review and Meta-Analyses of Randomised Controlled Trials and Cohort Studies." *BMJ* 346 (January 2013): e7492 doi:10.1136/bmj.e7492.

Wagner, M., M.P. Schlüsener, T.A. Ternes, and J. Oehlmann. "Identification of Putative Steroid Receptor Antagonists in Bottled Water: Combining Bioassays and High-Resolution Mass Spectrometry." *PLOS ONE* 8, no. 8 (August 2013):e72472. doi:10.1371/journal.pone.0072472.

Yang, Q. "Gain Weight by 'Going Diet'? Artificial Sweeteners and the Neurobiology of Sugar Cravings." *Yale Journal of Biology and Medicine* 83, no. 2 (June 2010): 101–108. Accessed February 10, 2016. www.ncbi.nlm.nih.gov/PMC/articles/PMC2892765.

Yang, Q., Z. Zhang, E.W. Gregg, D. Flanders, R. Merritt, and F.B. Hu. "Added Sugar Intake and Cardiovascular Diseases Mortality Among U.S. Adults." *JAMA Internal Medicine* 174, no. 4 (April 2014): 516–524. doi:10.1001/jamainternmed.2013.13563.

Chapter 13

Diamanti-Kandarakis, E., J-P. Bourguignon, L.C. Giudice, et al. "Endocrine-Disrupting Chemicals: An Endocrine Society Scientific Statement." *Endocrine Reviews* 30, no. 4 (June 2009): 293–342. doi:10.1210/er.2009-0002.

Chapter 15

Sebastian, R.S., C.W. Enns, and J.D. Goldman. "Snacking Patterns of U.S. Adults: What We Eat in America, NHANES 2007–2008." *Food Surveys Research Group Dietary Data Brief No. 4* June 2011. Accessed June 26, 2016. www.ars.usda.gov/SP2UserFiles/Place/80400530/pdf/DBrief/4_adult_snacking_0708.pdf.

Chapter 16

Wagner, M., M.P. Schlüsener, T.A. Ternes, and J. Oehlmann. "Identification of Putative Steroid Receptor Antagonists in Bottled Water: Combining Bioassays and High-Resolution Mass Spectrometry." *PLOS ONE, no.8.* (August 2013): e72472. Accessed April 6, 2016. doi:10.1371/journal.pone.0072472.

ACKNOWLEDGMENTS

There are so many people who have helped bring this book to fruition, and, to them, I'll be forever thankful.

First, my health coaching client Kerry Anderson, who, unbeknownst to her, planted the seeds of this book many years ago! After one of our initial meetings, she recounted how she spent an agonizing two hours at the grocery store, frustrated, trying to figure out what to buy, and how she wished someone would just give her a list of exactly what to choose . . . this book is it!

To Ivanka Trump, who has been an incredible supporter of my work over the years. Years ago, she watered those seeds when she graciously extended an invitation for me to take her entire team on a grocery store tour as part of a corporate wellness event and an invitation to be an entrepreneur-in-residence. I am grateful for her support in spreading the message of the importance of eating well for good health.

To Dean Ornish, a pioneer in the food and lifestyle-as-medicine space, for all your contributions to medicine and society, and for graciously writing the foreword to this book.

To all of my clients, whom I love so dearly, thank you for allowing me to be your guide over the years and for teaching me as much as I teach you. Especially those who I have personally led on grocery store tours—your questions have all (hopefully) made it into this book.

To Diana Chaplin, one of the first to read the initial iteration of what was to become this book, who encouraged me to get this published. To Julie Morris for being ever inspiring and introducing me to my agent. To my agent Marilyn Allen for her guidance and my editor Jill Alexander at Fair Winds Press for believing in me and this book! And to the whole Fair Winds team for making this book a reality.

To Doug Evans, thank you for all of your generosity, advice, and support. To my family, for always being there for me.

ABOUT THE AUTHOR

Maria Marlowe is an integrative nutrition health coach, author, and speaker. She inspires audiences, and she coaches individuals to reverse acne, lose weight, and improve their health through a real-food diet and by developing healthy habits that stick. Her website provides delicious healthy recipes, meal plans, and online programs. Maria graduated summa cum laude from Fordham University. Visit her at mariamarlowe.com, and on Instagram @mariamarlowe.

INDEX

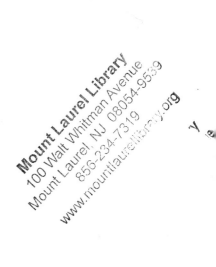